THE
FAT-LOSS
BLITZ

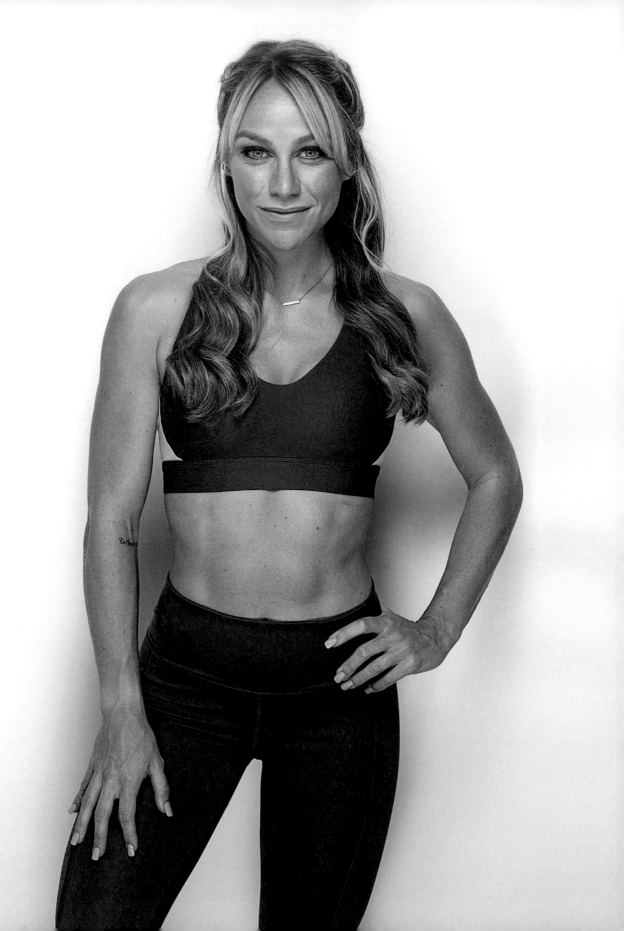

THE FAT-LOSS BLITZ
CHLOE MADELEY

Flexible diet and exercise plans
to transform your body –
whatever your fitness level

BANTAM PRESS

LONDON · NEW YORK · TORONTO · SYDNEY · AUCKLAND

TRANSWORLD PUBLISHERS
61–63 Uxbridge Road, London W5 5SA
www.penguin.co.uk

Transworld is part of the Penguin Random House group
of companies whose addresses can be found at global.
penguinrandomhouse.com

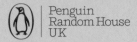
Penguin
Random House
UK

First published in Great Britain in 2018 by Bantam Press
an imprint of Transworld Publishers

Project editor: Jo Roberts-Miller
Design: Smith & Gilmour
Cover and exercise photography by Sam Riley
Food photography by Smith & Gilmour
Food styling by Vicki Keppel-Compton

A CIP catalogue record for this book is available from the
British Library.

ISBN 9781787630116

Typeset in Museo Slab 9.75/14pt
Printed and bound in Italy by Pi

Penguin Random House is com
our business, our readers and ou
Forest Stewardship Council® ce

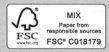
FSC
www.fsc.org
MIX
Paper from
responsible sources
FSC® C018179

1 3 5 7 9 10 8 6 4 2

The health and fitness information
in this book has been compiled by
way of general guidance in relation
to the specific subjects addressed.
It is not intended as a substitute
for medical advice. Please consult
your GP or healthcare professional
before performing the exercises
described in this book, particularly
if you are pregnant, elderly or
have chronic or recurring medical
conditions. Do not attempt any
of the exercises while under the
influence of alcohol or drugs.
Discontinue any exercise that
causes you pain or severe
discomfort and consult a medical
expert. So far as the author is aware
the information given is correct
and up to date at the time of
publication. The author and
publishers disclaim, as far as the
law allows, any liability arising
directly or indirectly from the use,
or misuse, of the information
contained in this book.

CONTENTS

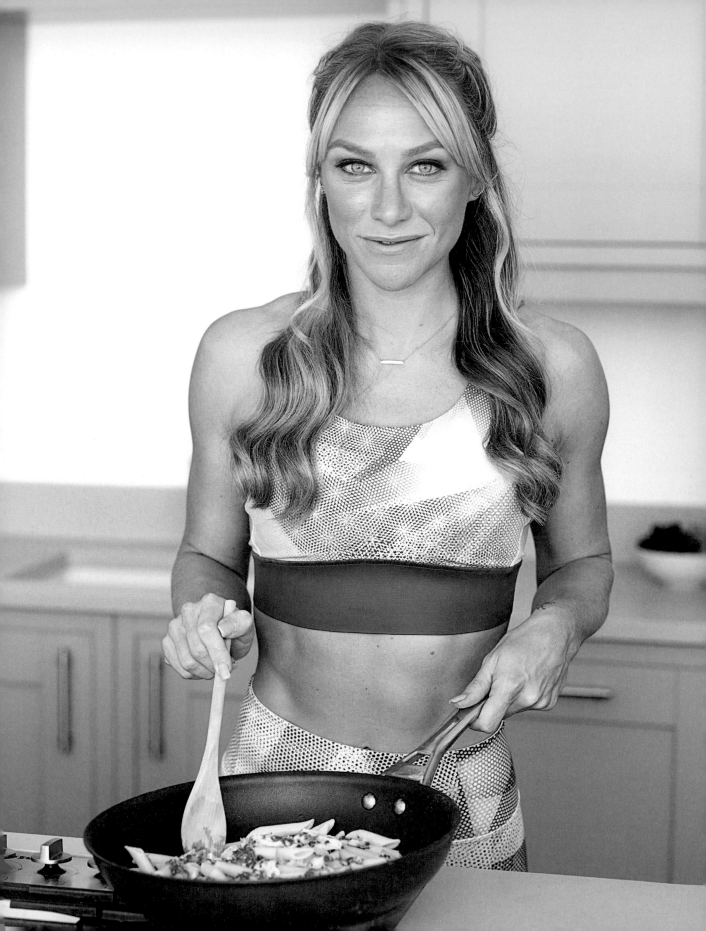

INTRODUCTION

Dearest Blitzers both new and old,
Welcome to *The Fat-Loss Blitz*!

I want to start by saying a big fat thank you to those of you who bought my first book. Your initial trust and support, subsequent dedication and commitment, and phenomenal before and after photos have given me the opportunity to write this follow-up book, and I am so very grateful to you all.

First and foremost, *The Fat-Loss Blitz* is *not* just my last book with a new cover and subtitle slapped on the front of it.

Since the release of *The 4-Week Body Blitz*, I have continued to learn more in my own field and I have continued to learn more from you. The scientific understanding of the body is ever-evolving. New studies are being released constantly, counter studies usually follow, and professionals continue to raise new questions, begin new trials and find new answers.

The best personal trainers, coaches, nutritionists and doctors are the ones who read, watch, listen, trial and read some more, constantly reassessing and redeveloping their methods.

I'm not saying, 'Forget what you learned on *The 4-Week Body Blitz*!' because that defeats the *entire process* of learning. There were some great fundamental lessons to take away from that plan. But I *do* want to say, 'Trust *this* book 100%!' I have spent *a lot* of time watching your results, listening to your feedback, reading new studies, questioning my coaching heroes and bettering my knowledge on your behalf.

I've been chomping at the bit to write something new that I feel will be *even more* helpful than the original book, and while *The Fat-Loss Blitz* is designed to get you the same results as the original Blitz (fat loss and body transformation), the methods are different...

First, you now have *options...* There are three plans, tailored according to your level of fitness, so that Blitzers at different stages can all achieve their aesthetic goals:

The Sedentary Plan

The Active Plan

The Gym Plan

Each plan will follow the same overall *methods*, but with different diet and training instructions.

While the overall methods are always going to be the same for fat loss (a calorie deficit achieved via diet and training), an experienced weightlifter is going to need to implement a very different dietary *structure* to a complete beginner.

If you can be bothered to read the entire book from cover to cover, doing so will help your understanding of the general rules of health, fitness, nutrition, training and results but, if not, you can just find the right plan for you and focus on that.

Let's get started …

BEFORE YOU BEGIN...

There's something we need to talk about.

What is your recent diet and training history?

If you have been on any kind of diet for a while now and you can no longer get your body to respond, that means you have temporarily floored your hormone levels and metabolic rate, and you need to reset them. This will take a few weeks but it is both necessary for your *health* and imperative for aesthetic *results*.

If this sounds like you, stop whatever diet you are on *immediately*. You're going to be 'intuitive eating' for 4–12 weeks *before* beginning *The Fat-Loss Blitz*. The longer you can give your body to recover from whatever diet you have been on, the better. 'Diet breaks' typically last anywhere from a few weeks to a few months. I encourage you to use your intuition to determine how long you need.

Intuitive eating means:

>> Eating a balance of *healthy* protein, fat and carb sources at *every* meal (chicken, nuts, rice and veg, for example).

>> Eating no less than 3 big or 6 small meals a day.

>> Looking at food in terms of your *internal* physical *health* instead of how it will make you *look*.

>> Allowing yourself the odd day/ night off to *relax!*

Finally, when you are on your diet break, I want you to decrease your training, so you are exercising no more than 4 days a week for 1 hour a session.

Yes, you may gain some weight and, yes, you may gain some body fat, but guess what? You will be happy, you will be healthy and, eventually, you will be *ready* to achieve the results that have been escaping you for so long.

If you track calories and macros

Take a look at your numbers... Make sure you are hitting:

>> 2g protein per kg bodyweight

>> 1g carb per kg bodyweight

>> 1g fat per kg bodyweight

If you're not, work your way up to those numbers before starting a plan.

Then, each week, I want you to add 30g carbohydrates (120kcals) to your intake, until you are close to around 2000kcals a day.

Once there, I want you to stay put for at least 4–12 weeks to allow your body to both recover and readjust. Also, you should allow yourself the odd day/night off from tracking and relax.

THE TRAINING PLANS

How do you know which plan is right for you?

1. The Sedentary Plan

You should begin here if you are:

>> Unfit

>> Unsure

>> Inexperienced

>> Out of shape

>> In recovery (from illness/injury)

This section includes its own dietary instructions and a very gentle yet progressive 4-week training guide (see pages 54–67).

2. The Active Plan

You should begin here if you:

>> Enjoy regular (weekly) exercise but don't take it too seriously

>> Take part in sporadic gym classes/ online workouts/PT sessions/weekly runs/outdoor activities/group sports/ gym training

>> Want to continue with the exercises you already do and enjoy, but get the best results possible while doing so

This section includes its own dietary instructions and various suggestions and options in the 4-week training guide (see pages 70–91).

3. The Gym Plan

You should begin here if you:

>> Know how to train properly (resistance training/free weights/plyometrics/HIIT)

>> Take training seriously

>> Train often (4–6 days a week)

>> Want to get the absolute best results from your training and nutrition

This section includes its own dietary instructions and a gym-based, progressive 4-week training guide (see pages 94–157).

FAQ

When *The 4-Week Body Blitz* came out, readers contacted me on
a near daily basis, all with very similar questions. Often, they wanted
to start the plan but were hesitant as to whether or not it was right for
them. Here are some of the most common questions I was asked.
I hope that my answers will help you determine the suitability
of *The Fat-Loss Blitz* to your life.

Can men do *The Fat-Loss Blitz*?

Yes! I know I am a high-pitched,
screeching, blonde girl, but I have many
male clients. On top of that, fat loss is fat
loss. The only difference between a fat-loss
plan for a man and a fat-loss plan for a
woman is that men require a slightly
higher calorie count – details of which
I explain fully in each plan.

I have diabetes/health problems/ hormonal problems – can I follow the plan?

You'll need to speak to your doctor/
dietician/endocrinologist before starting
any diet or training plan. He or she will
either green light it, red light it, or adapt
it to suit you.

Can I follow the plan if I am older/ injured/unfit?

Yes! That is the beauty of this book –
there are plans to suit all fitness levels.

Can vegetarians/vegans/gluten freebies do this plan?

As long as you include the following
in your diet:

>> A complete protein source (e.g. soy)
>> A fat source (e.g. avocado)
>> A carb source (e.g. rice)

You can do *any* of my plans.

Do I have to start tracking/stop tracking calories and macros on *The Fat-Loss Blitz*?

You can follow a plan and never track
a thing because this book has meal
plans and is *not* an IIFYM (If It Fits Your
Macros) plan. However, if you *do* track
and you want to continue to do so, feel
free to use my nutrition plan alongside
MyFitnessPal or whatever app you use,
and manipulate your specific intakes
to hit your required numbers
throughout the day.

What if I don't like a particular food?

You don't have to eat any food you don't like on *The Fat-Loss Blitz*. You can swap any protein, fat or carb in any of your meals or recipes by using The Food Bible (see page 22). For example, you could swap tuna for chicken (protein), avocado for eggs (fat), or a small jacket potato for a small bowl of pasta (carbohydrate).

Why don't my Build Your Own Meal macros look like your recipe macros?

Every instruction in The Food Bible and every meal in the recipe section has been calculated to hit the same calorie count. Macros will differ slightly from meal to meal, but the overall macro *methods* are maintained throughout. For example, if I tell you to pick a portion of protein, a portion of carb and a portion of veg for your lunch, or if I tell you to pick a high-carb recipe for your lunch, they will each total the same calories. The recipe might contain slightly more fat than a meal that you build, but the calories and macro *methods* will be the same.

Does it matter when I eat my snacks and/or meals?

Eat *whenever* you fancy eating. For example, feel free to add one of your snacks into your lunch, or eat your snacks together before bed. As long as you eat everything I tell you to eat – nothing more, nothing less – you can eat it *whenever* suits you best. *However*, I do want you to eat one of your *meals* as soon as possible post exercise (ideally within the hour).

Can I follow this plan if I am pregnant?

While you can continue your usual training plan if you are pregnant, you cannot start a new body transformation plan. One body transformation at a time.

Can I follow this plan post-natal?

As soon as you get the all-clear from your doctor, you can do *The Fat-Loss Blitz*.

Can I do *The Fat-Loss Blitz* when breastfeeding?

Yes, but bear in mind that you burn anywhere up to 500kcals a day breastfeeding, so if you track calories and macros you need to make up for this. If you don't track, add in another meal and snack to your intake each day, ideally around your training.

I am on week 1 and feeling headachy/dizzy – is this normal?

Yes, week 1 can be tough because of sugar withdrawals. Unfortunately, it is unavoidable for some of us and you just have to power through to week 2. If it gets particularly bad, eat a piece of fruit or drink some fruit juice in order to pick up your blood sugar levels quickly.

Can I have a breakfast for dinner or a lunch for breakfast?

As long as you are following your dietary instructions (in terms of carbs or fats), you can absolutely have brunch or brinner!

You say I should always try to include non-starchy veg in my meals and/or snacks, but I'm having yoghurt for breakfast, so how do I do this?

Try to include non-starchy veg in as many meals as you can. Non-starchy veg are essential for our overall health. They contain *micronutrients,* AKA vitamins and minerals, not to mention other pivotal substances, such as fibre. They are also very low in calories and, owing to their fibre content, will keep you feeling fuller for longer, so *try* to get them in whenever and wherever you can. But if you can't always manage it, that's OK, too.

Can I go out to eat on this plan?

Yes, you just need to make sure what you eat fits in with the plan. For example, a low-carb meal would be a portion of protein and a portion of veg (the butter or oil used to cook it would count towards your fats). This could be a tuna steak and veg, or a big chicken salad. A high carb meal would be a portion of protein and a carb. For example, sushi rolls or roast chicken and roast potatoes.

Do I have to be a gym member to do this plan?

No. The Sedentary Plan is *extremely* straightforward in terms of becoming fit and active. The Active Plan is extremely flexible with regard to what exercises you do and when. Even the Gym Plan can be edited to work with your own resources, if you have weights at home.

I've been on the diet for a few days/weeks now and I feel bloated/gassy – why?

This is probably down to one of two things:

›› Cruciferous vegetables (broccoli/cauliflower/cabbage)
›› Whey protein powders/bars

A lot of people struggle with one or both of the above. If you find excessive bloating or gas is starting to occur, cut one from your diet for a few days. Reintroduce it *in small quantities* once your symptoms have eased and see how you respond. I am hesitant to tell somebody to cut something from their diet *completely* and *forever* because this can often make an intolerance worse. However, if you *have* to, then do.

I have weights at home – can I implement them into this plan?

Yes, absolutely! If you are doing a circuit that has, say, a squat, then by all means make this a weighted squat.

What weights should I lift?

I cannot tell you what weight to lift as it is 100% subjective and depends on *your own* strength. A weight that challenges me would do absolutely nothing for my partner. A weight that challenges a beginner would probably do nothing for me. Everybody is different. I want you to choose a weight that allows you to complete every set, but that leaves you really struggling by the last few reps.

Why do I feel weaker/more tired today than I did yesterday?

The calorie deficit in this plan is effective, but it's not so extreme that you'll struggle to train. However, *any* calorie deficit, especially when coupled with a new training plan, is going to see you having tired days. It's just the way it is. Tired days can also be a direct result of fat loss. Try to fight on through and embrace the experience for what it is. However, if you have to take a rest day or two consecutively at any point, then listen to your body and accept that's what you have to do.

Can I do a plan as well as my X/ instead of my Y/alongside my Z?

Yes! The beauty of *The Fat-Loss Blitz* is that it is a lot less rigid in terms of what you can do and don't have to do than the original *Body Blitz*. So long as you stick to the times and intensities I instruct, you can swap one of my sessions for your favourite team sport or a session in the pool.

This may sound like lazy advice, but when it comes to your diet, training and physical responses, a lot of common sense and intuition is required. Obviously I want you to stick to the plan, but I also want you to listen to your body... If you need a rest day, take one. If it's your birthday and you want a glass of champagne, drink a glass of champagne!

SLEEP AND REST

Now I want to talk about the flip side of exercise – sleep and rest – and how equally important they are...

Rest, recovery and sleep are going to play a *huge* role in both your enjoyment of this process *and* your aesthetic results. On the scales, in the mirror, during workouts and even during work hours, you are going to feel, look, act and perform a hell of a lot better if you are well rested and well recovered.

If at any point you feel like you need an added day off training, take one – just try to get right back on track with your plan the next day.

However, if you feel you need more than one day off, you can take two consecutive days to rest and recover. You will probably find that you both look and feel a lot better once you do.

When it comes to sleep, I want you to *try* to get eight hours of sleep a night. I know this may be exceptionally hard for those of you with young children and/or a demanding job, but try, try and try again. You might just surprise yourself...

The sympathetic and parasympathetic states are equally important to one another. Your body appreciates a big, old push every now and then, but it also appreciates a big, old rest. Like all things in life, you need to be conscious of balance. Try to train yourself to come in and out of these two states quickly through breathing, resting and recovery techniques.

CONTINUATION AND PROGRESSION

Once you have completed one of the 4-week plans, you can continue for up to 24 weeks (6 months) in total if you wish. You can do this by remaining on the plan you started with, or by progressing on to the next...

For example, if you complete the Sedentary Plan and want to progress to the Active Plan, then this would be a great thing to do. However, you could just follow the Sedentary Plan for up to 24 weeks.

The same rule applies to the Active Plan: you can continue with this plan for up to 24 weeks, or progress to the Gym Plan.

Finally, if you are on the Gym Plan, you can follow this for up to 24 weeks.

After 24 weeks, though, I would encourage you to reverse out of diet and training *slowly*, week by week, until you get to a level you are happy and comfortable with.

You can do this by:

>> Adding 1 carb meal (or snack) to your daily intake each week

>> Completing 1 less training session each week *or* gradually decreasing your training times each week

Continue to do this, week by week, until you reach a level you are personally happy and comfortable with.

When it comes to my long-term diet and training advice, I normally recommend:

>> Protein and carbs pre- and post-training

>> Protein and fats the rest of the time

>> Omnipresent vegetables

>> Training no less than 4 times a week and no more than 6 times

>> Training for no longer than 1 hour per occasion

>> Relaxed days/nights off without guilt when physically and/or socially necessary

While I don't want you to *push* your body for more than 24 weeks, I also don't want you to become sedentary and/or overeat afterwards.

You should always aim to find a good balance of activity and rest, healthy eating, and lenience. *All* are important for your overall mental *and* physical health.

Balance looks different for everyone, but make sure you monitor yourself and don't let it get either side of the extreme.

After a few months of a more relaxed approach, if you want to try *The Fat-Loss Blitz* again, it will be just as effective, if not more so.

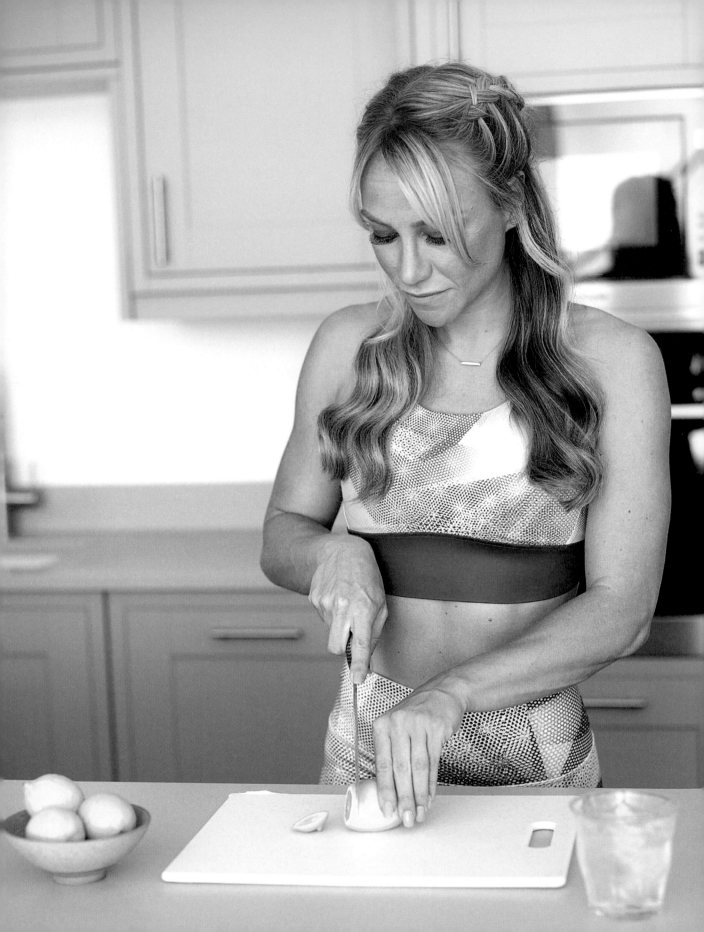

THE NUTRITION PLAN

THE NUTRITION PLAN IS SPLIT INTO TWO SECTIONS:

1. The Food Bible (see pages 22–39)
2. Recipes (see pages 159–213)

Feel free to use The Food Bible to build your own meals *and/or* cook from the recipes I've provided.

Once you've decided which plan to follow, you will find your *specific* nutrition instructions there. The nutrition plan found on these pages is a base that everyone can use, whichever plan you are on.

Those of you who know my original book will notice that The Food Bible is not nearly as strict, and that there are *lots* of fun new options here – including cheese! That is because *this time*, I decided that, even though you will not feel as full from a portion of cheese as you will from a portion of eggs, whether to eat cheese or eggs is a decision you can make for yourself. I've gone to great lengths to calculate all calorie and macro values to give you more choice.

However, you'll see that *some* things are still not permitted – cakes, croissants and crêpes, for example, are so high in calories that there is just no room for them, unless you sacrifice a significant amount of food elsewhere. If you notice that something is *not* included in The Food Bible, this is why.

You should also be aware that, for example, two pork sausages may have roughly the same *macros* and *calories* as a fillet of salmon, but it goes without saying that the salmon is *far* better for you from a health perspective.

You probably already knew that, but you might not know *why*...

Put simply, while a calorie is a calorie, a carb is a carb, a protein is a protein and a fat is a fat, there are different subcategories, and some are far healthier than others.

Carbohydrates can be refined sugars (sweets and juice) or starches (grains and potatoes). So, while a packet of sweets here and there is *not* going to make you fat (*no* single food 'makes you fat'), one packet of sweets is going to be the same number of calories as three bowls of oats... that's one snack traded in for three small meals.

Proteins can be made up of *essential* amino acids (e.g. meat) or *non-essential* amino acids (e.g. nuts). *Essential* amino acids will *always* be a better option as our body does not naturally make these, yet it desperately needs them, which is why they are *essential*.

However, our bodies *do* make non-essential amino acids, therefore they are *non-essential* in our diets.

Fats can be *essential* fatty acids (e.g. oily fish) or *non-essential* fatty acids (e.g. red meats). While we do actually need *both*, we need *essential* fatty acids a lot more, so fish is usually a better source of dietary fat.

There are nutritious calories (food) and wasted calories (alcohol) – you can eat a 300-calorie meal or drink a few glasses of wine but, ideally, you want your 300 calories to satiate you, benefit your body and encourage your body transformation results.

What I'm trying to say is that there is no such thing as a 'good' or 'bad' food. However, there *is* such a thing as a *more satiating* and/or *healthier* food.

If you want body transformation, specifically, your primary concerns should be:

>> Calories
>> Macronutrients
>> Health

Try to tick every box, but don't panic if you have to be (or simply want to be) a bit more flexible from time to time.

Healthy eating should always be your primary concern – we all want to live long, happy, healthy lives. However, never be fooled – body transformation is a science. Calories in (food) versus calories out (movement) will determine your weight gain or weight loss.

THE FOOD BIBLE

The Food Bible is made up of information
about the 3 macronutrients that will
constitute your weekly diet:

1. Protein

2. Fat

3. Carbohydrate

Every food has been calorie- and macro-calculated
and matched, allowing users to swap one option
for another when and where necessary.

For example, if you don't like tuna, you can
have chicken (protein).

If you don't like avocado, you can have eggs (fats).

If you don't like bread, you can have oats (carbs).

This can be done when following the recipes, too.
If you want to make the Tortilla Pizza (see page 194)
with prawns instead of chicken sausages, then
go right ahead! Just swap the macros:
2 chicken sausages = 100g prawns.

1. PROTEIN

Protein should always be your dominant macro when following *The Fat-loss Blitz*, no matter which plan you are on. It should be the staple macro for all your daily meals and snacks.

All proteins marked in **red** are higher calorie owing to a higher fat content. If you choose one of these as your protein source, it will *also* be your fat source for that meal.

Anything in **green** is a personal brand suggestion. These suggestions are not endorsed – they are simply based on my years of tracking calories and macros and finding the most 'bang for my buck' foods.

PROTEIN	EASE	MEASURE
15% Beef Mince	150g packet	150g
10% Beef Mince	175g packet	175g
5% Beef Mince	200g packet	200g
Chicken (skinless/boneless)	1 breast	Approx. 125g
Chicken Chipolatas Heck Chicken Chipolatas	3	
Cod	1 small fillet	Approx. 150g
Crayfish	1 small packet	Typically 150g
Duck (skinless/boneless)	1 small breast	Approx. 125g

PROTEIN	EASE	MEASURE
EatLean Protein Cheese		80g
Eggs	2 small OR 4 small	
Egg Whites	8 large	Approx. 300g
Fillet Steak	1 small steak	Approx. 200g
Haddock	1 small fillet	Approx. 120g
King Scallops	2 large	Approx. 120g
Lobster	1 small lobster	
Mussels	1 small bowl	Approx. 150g
Plain Fat-free Cottage Cheese	200g tub	200g
Plain Full-fat Cottage Cheese	200g tub	200g
Plain 0% Greek Yoghurt Fage	200g tub	200g
Plain Full-fat Greek Yoghurt Fage	200g tub	200g
Plain Soy Yogurt	300g tub	300g
Pork Bacon	2 slices	
Pork Sausage	1 sausage OR 2 sausages	

PROTEIN	EASE	MEASURE
Prawns	1 small packet	Approx. 150g
Quorn (mince/pieces)	100g	100g
Salmon Fillet	1 small fillet	Approx. 120g
Scallops	1 small packet/bowl	Typically 150g
Smoked Salmon	4 small slices	Approx. 80g
Sole	1 small fillet	Approx. 150g
Soy (Tofu etc)	1 packet	Typically 100g
Squid	1 small packet/bowl	Typically 150g
Tinned Salmon	1 small tin	Typically 105g
Tinned Tuna (in water or brine)	1 tin	Typically 110g (drained weight)
Tinned Tuna (in sunflower or olive oil)	1 tin	Typically 110g (drained weight)
Tuna Steak	1 small steak	Approx. 120g
Turkey (skinless/boneless)	1 small breast	Approx. 125g
Turkey Bacon	3 slices	
Turkey Breast Mince	1 packet	Typically 100g
Vegan Protein Powder MYPROTEIN Vegan Blend	1 scoop	Typically 25–30g
Whey Protein Powder PhD Diet Whey	1 scoop	Typically 25–30g

2. FATS

Your daily fat intake will depend on which plan you are following.

All fats marked in **red** are higher calorie owing to a higher protein content. If you choose one of these as your fat source, it will *also* be your protein source for that meal.

All **green** notes are my personal brand suggestions. These suggestions are not endorsed – they are simply based on my years of tracking calories and macros and finding the most 'bang for my buck' foods.

FAT	EASE	MEASURE
15% Beef Mince	150g packet	150g
10% Beef Mince	175g packet	175g
5% Beef Mince	200g packet	200g
Almond Butter Meridian	1 level tbsp	Approx. 15g
Avocado	½ small avocado	Approx. 60g
Brie	2 knife smears	Approx. 40g
Butter	1 level tbsp	15g
Cacao Nibs MYPROTEIN	1 level tbsp	Approx. 15g
Camembert	2 knife smears	Approx. 40g
Cashew Butter Meridian	1 level tbsp	Approx. 15g

FAT	EASE	MEASURE
Cheddar	1 small handful, grated	Approx. 30g
Dark Chocolate (90% cocoa solids)	2 squares	25g
Double Cream	2 level tbsp	Approx. 30ml
Edam Cheese	1 small handful, grated	Approx. 30g
Eggs	2 small OR 4 small	
Emmental	1 small handful, grated	Approx. 30g
Feta Cheese	1 small handful, crumbled	Approx. 30g
Fillet Steak	1 small steak	Approx. 200g
Full fat Cottage Cheese	100g tub OR 200g tub	100g OR 200g
Full-fat Cream Cheese	2 level tbsp	Approx. 30g
Halloumi	1 slice	Typically 30g
Hummus	2 level tbsp	Approx. 30g
Mayonnaise	1 level tbsp	Approx. 15g
Mozzarella	2 small handfuls, torn or grated	Approx. 60g
Nuts (all)	1 small palm size	Approx. 20g
Oil (all)	1 level tbsp	15ml
Olives (all)	1 good handful	Approx. 75g

FAT	EASE	MEASURE
Parmesan	2 level tbsp	Approx. 20g
Peanut Butter Meridian	1 level tbsp	Approx. 15g
Pesto (all)	1 level tbsp	Approx. 15g
Plain Full-fat Greek Yoghurt Fage	100g tub OR 200g tub	100g OR 200g
Pork Bacon	2 slices	Approx. 30g
Salmon Fillet	1 small fillet	Approx. 120g
Seeds (all)	1 level tbsp	Approx. 15g
Single Cream	4 level tbsp	Approx. 60ml
Smoked Salmon	4 slices	Approx. 80g
Soured Cream	4 level tbsp	Approx. 60ml
Tahini Meridian	1 level tbsp	Approx. 15g
Tinned Salmon	1 tin	105g
Tinned Tuna (in sunflower or olive oil)	1 tin	110g (drained weight)

3. CARBOHYDRATES

Your daily carb intake will depend on which plan you are following.

All **green** notes are my personal brand suggestions. These suggestions are not endorsed – they are simply based on my years of tracking calories and macros and finding the most 'bang for my buck' foods.

CARBOHYDRATE	EASE	MEASURE
Bread (wholegrain)	1 slice	Approx. 40–50g
Couscous	1 small bowl	Approx. 40g (dry weight) Approx. 100g (cooked weight)
Crumpet (any)	1 normal OR 2 thins	Approx. 55g OR Approx. 50g
English Muffin	1 small	Approx. 60g
Fruit (any)	1 small portion	Approx. 50g
Honey	2 level tbsp	Approx. 30g
Legumes (all pulses: beans/ peas/lentils etc.)	¼ tin	Approx. 100g
Pasta (wholegrain)	1 small bowl	Approx. 40g (dry weight) Approx. 80g (cooked weight)

CARBOHYDRATE	EASE	MEASURE
Pitta Bread (wholegrain)	1 standard size	Approx. 50g
Plain Bagel (wholegrain)	½ normal OR 1 thin	Approx. 45g OR Approx. 45g
Plain Granola	1 handful	Approx. 30g (dry weight)
Plain Muesli	1 small bowl	Approx. 30g (dry weight)
Plain Oats (any)	3 level tbsp OR 1 small bowl	Approx. 30g (dry weight)
Plain Popcorn	1 small bag OR 2 large handfuls OR 25g kernels	Approx. 25g Approx. 25g 25g
Plain Rice Cakes	3 rice cakes	Approx. 30g
Plain Puffed Rice Cereal (any)	1 small bowl	Approx. 30g (dry weight)
Plain Small American Pancake/ Scotch Pancake	1 small	Approx. 40g
Plain Small Tortilla Wrap (wholegrain)	1 small	Approx. 40g
Plain Wheat Biscuits Weetabix	2 biscuits	Approx. 40g

CARBOHYDRATE	EASE	MEASURE
Potato (+ all starchy veg: parsnips/plantain/pumpkin/green peas/corn etc.)	1 small serving	Approx. 150g
Quinoa	1 small bowl	Approx. 40g (dry weight) Approx. 100g (cooked weight)
Rice (wholegrain)	1 small bowl	Approx. 40g (dry weight) Approx. 80g (cooked weight)
Taco Shells	2 shells	Approx. 15g each

It's really important to accept that if you *want* results, you can't be laissez-faire with portion sizes. You may think that a heaped tablespoon, as opposed to a level tablespoon, won't make a difference, but it will double or even triple the calories of that serving, taking you out of a calorie deficit and into a calorie surplus. Follow the instructions and you will see the results!

VEGETABLES

Try to include non-starchy vegetables in all of your meals as they are essential for both internal and external good health.

Vegetables contain micronutrients, AKA vitamins and minerals, not to mention other pivotal substances, such as fibre. They are very low calorie and, owing to their high fibre content, will keep you feeling fuller for longer.

I have listed the most common non-starchy veg. However, if there are any missing from the list, the same rules about portion size still apply.

1 portion = 1 large handful

>> All green leaves (lettuce/spinach/rocket etc.)

>> Asparagus

>> Aubergine

>> Bean sprouts

>> Beetroot

>> Broccoli

>> Cabbage (savoy/white/red/kale/Brussels sprouts/pak choi etc.)

>> Cauliflower

>> Celery

>> Courgette

>> Cucumber (fresh/pickled etc.)

>> Green beans

>> Leeks

>> Mushrooms (any)

>> Okra

>> Onions (white/red/pickled etc)

>> Peppers (any)

>> Radishes

>> Tomatoes (cherry/vine/plum/chopped/tinned/passata etc.)

ADDITIONS TO MEALS AND SNACKS

I've said it before and I'll say it again – your meals and/or snacks do *not* have to be bland!

Feel free to use any of the ingredients listed below in or alongside your meals and/or snacks.

All **green** notes are my personal brand suggestions. These suggestions are not endorsed – they are simply based on my years of tracking calories and macros and finding the most 'bang for my buck' foods.

ADDITIONS TO MEALS

>> 1 clove garlic/1 tsp chopped garlic

>> 1 tsp gravy granules (any)

>> 1 tsp hot sauce Tabasco

>> 1 tsp lemon/lime juice

>> 1 tsp mustard (any)

>> 1 tsp MYPROTEIN Sugar-free Syrup (any)

>> 1 tsp reduced sugar ketchup Heinz 50% Less Sugar/Salt Ketchup

>> 1 tsp soy sauce (any)

>> 1 stock cube (any)

>> 1 tsp Sweet Freedom Choc Shot

>> 1 tsp vinegar (any)

>> chilli peppers (any)

>> Fry Light cooking spray (any)

>> salt/pepper/herbs/spices

>> MYPROTEIN FlavDrops (any)

DIET FOODS

I am a big believer in eating clean, healthy, single-ingredient wholefoods. Not only are they better in terms of *health*, they are also a lot more satiating in terms of *hunger*.

However, I would be lying if I said I didn't use the odd trick to help with adherence.

All the diet foods listed below are ones that I have found helpful over the years. I've included advice on how to use them.

All **green** notes are my personal brand suggestions. These suggestions are not endorsed – they are simply based on my years of tracking calories and macros and finding the most 'bang for my buck' foods.

FOOD	PORTION	INSTRUCTION
Hartley's 10 Cal Jelly (any)	1 tub (typically 175g)	1 tub daily alongside meal/snack
Lo-Dough	1 piece	1 piece daily to replace veg in 1 meal
MYPROTEIN's My Bar Zero protein bars (any)	1 bar	1 bar daily to count as 2 snacks
Skinny Cow's Mint Double Choc Lolly	1 lolly	1 daily to replace 1 carb option
Zero Noodles OR Barenaked Rice/Noodles	1 packet	1 daily alongside meal/snack

DRINKS

I want *everyone* who follows this book to be *aiming* to drink 4 litres of water *daily*.

What I learned from my first book was that *a lot* of people struggle to hit this amount at the beginning of the plan. So, taking this into account, please feel free to work your way up to drinking 4 litres as the weeks progress.

Allow yourself a couple of hot drinks in the morning, while sipping on a 1-litre bottle of water into the early afternoon. Repeat this process mid-afternoon into early evening and, hey presto, you have achieved your water intake for the day

Below is a list of the drinks, in addition to water, that you are allowed to consume on this plan...

Drinks marked in **blue** count towards your daily water intake

DRINK	PORTION
Caffeinated Hot Drinks (Tea/Coffee etc.)	Up to 2 daily (morning/afternoon)
Decaffeinated Hot Drinks (Decaffeinated Coffee/Herbal Tea etc.)	Unlimited
Diet Drinks	1 daily
Skimmed Milk Unsweetened Almond Milk Unsweetened Coconut Milk Unsweetend Soy Milk Unsweetened Cashew Milk	1 tbsp to be used in your 2 daily caffeinated hot drinks

MY FAVOURITE SNACKS

You'll see that daily snacks are allowed and essential for each of the 4-week plans.

Your snack will either be a protein or a carbohydrate (depending on your plan and/or day) and you are free to choose anything you want from The Food Bible according to which macro is required. As long as you follow the portion sizes correctly, you can choose *any* protein or carb option you like – see the tables on pages 23–25 and 29–31. If you need some help with snack ideas, though, here are some of my favourites. But don't worry – you don't have to stick to these.

CARBOHYDRATE SNACK OPTIONS

CARBOHYDRATE	EASE	MEASURE
Fruit (any)	1 small portion	Approx. 50g
Hartley's 10 Cal Jelly (any)	1 tub	Typically 175g 1 tub daily alongside meal/snack
Plain Popcorn	1 small bag OR 2 large handfuls OR 25g kernels	Approx. 25g Approx. 25g 25g kernels
Plain Rice Cakes	3 rice cakes	Approx. 30g
Skinny Cow's Mint Double Choc Lolly	1 lolly	1 daily to replace 1 carb option

PROTEIN SNACK OPTIONS

PROTEIN	EASE	MEASURE
Eggs	2 small	
MYPROTEIN's My Bar Zero protein bars (any)	1 bar	1 bar daily to count as 2 snacks
Plain 0% Greek Yoghurt Fage	200g tub	200g
Plain Fat-free Cottage Cheese	200g tub	200g
Plain Soy Yoghurt	300g tub	300g
Soy (Tofu etc)	1 packet	Typically 100g
Whey Protein Powder PhD Diet Whey	1 scoop	Typically 25–30g
Vegan Protein Powder MYPROTEIN Vegan Blend	1 scoop	Typically 25–30g

SUPPLEMENTS

I try to get 100% of my nutrition from the food I eat but there are benefits to taking a few specific supplements as well.

Please keep in mind that you *do not need* to take *any* supps in order to see progress.

However, as I said, I feel there are benefits to a small few.

Here are my recommendations:

❯❯ *Protein Supplements*
I have a sweet tooth and protein is my dominant macro, no matter what phase I am in (fat loss or muscle building). Because of this, I usually have one protein supplement a day, be it a bar or a powder – usually immediately post-workout to get some protein in my body ASAP or I make a protein mug cake late at night (see my Chocolate Almond Protein Cake page 172).

Try to go for the lower calorie, lower carb and lower fat protein supps that have a good hit of whey (which is a *great* complete protein source).

I like to use PhD Diet Whey as it tastes great, has easy-to-fit macros and is perfect to cook with. In terms of bars, Myprotein's My Bar Zero bars have great macro counts (one of these bars would equal two snacks on all the plans in this book).

❯❯ *Multivitamins/Vitamin C*
Take multivits every day after breakfast. Training and dieting can take a bit of a toll on your body – a lot of people find they are more susceptible to illness in the first few weeks of a new plan. So do everything you can to ward this off – drink water, eat greens and take your multivits.

❯❯ *Omega Oils*
I take omega oils daily after all my meals. They reduce inflammation (which is perfect for those who exercise) and support organ health. I saw my digestion improve when I began taking them, too. In my opinion, these supps are a daily must.

❯❯ *Probiotics*
You can take probiotics in drink, food or pill form. I take the latter to avoid blowing my calories and macros, and I strongly suggest that you do, too.

Probiotics will take care of your digestive system and immune system simultaneously, a must for your everyday life, but *especially* when starting a new diet and exercise plan.

A few weeks after I started taking probiotics I saw my bloat disappear and my results finally shone through.

Start small – don't go for something extra strength and don't exceed the recommended dosage as your GI tract can take a little while to adjust to probiotics.

>> BCAAs (Branch Chain Amino Acids)

BCAAs (branch chain amino acids – AKA complete proteins) are appropriate for those who perform resistance training *and* cardio together. Pre-, intra- and/or post-workout, this supplement can help protect your muscle when you're working at 100%. It will also optimise recovery.

They're also a great option for those of you who like sugary drinks, as they come in flavoured powder form to mix with water.

>> Creatine

This supplement is ideal for those who lift heavy weights. Creatine can give your muscles that added oomph when it comes to training, improving high-intensity performance and encouraging muscle growth

This is *not* a steroid and it will *not* make you 'bulky'. It is a substance that occurs naturally in our bodies and taking a daily supplement of creatine can improve your strength training.

>> Caffeine

A strong cup of coffee will do just as well as a supplement, but if you want to try a pre-workout, then go for it.

However, if you can find one that has been tested by Informed-Sport (a global quality assurance programme for sports nutrition products), you're reducing the risk of a crazy buzz pre workout (it may *sound* fun but, believe me, it does *not* give you a better training session!).

The effects and bioavailability of supplements are constantly being reevaluated and called into question. I used to read nothing but negative press about multivits, but after I did a bit of scientific digging, I came to the conclusion that they are, in fact, incredibly beneficial. If you are interested in learning more about supplements and their benefits, I highly recommend following Dr Rhonda Patrick.

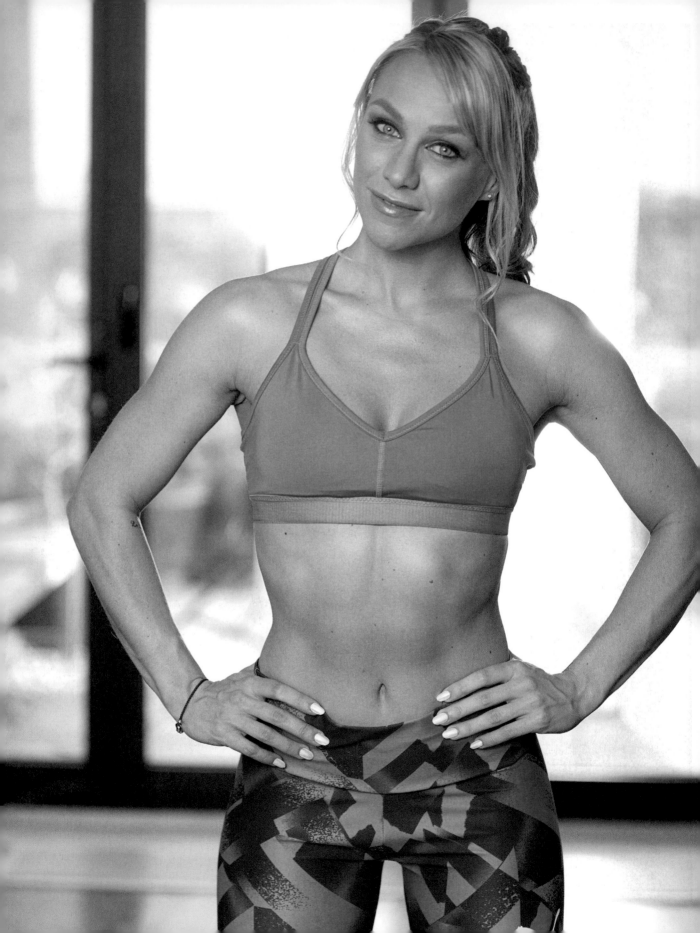

STRETCHING

You *must* warm up before and cool
down after every training session.

Think of your body as a piece of chewing
gum – if it's cold and you bend it,
it will snap. If it's warm and you bend it,
it will be supple and move.

Please note:
Warm-up stretches are performed
dynamically, meaning with a slow
and gentle bouncy movement.

To make a stretch dynamic, hold the
position and perform a gentle bounce
as you do so, for 8–10 repetitions.

Cool down stretches are performed
statically, meaning still.

To make a stretch static, hold the
position still for 8–10 seconds.

Some of the stretches are for warming
up only, most are for both warming up
and cooling down. All the stretches are
labelled so you know which are which.

SHOULDER STRETCH

WARM UP ONLY Stand up straight with your feet hip-width apart. Let your arms hang down by your sides. Place one hand across your body, rest it gently on the opposite side of your chest. In a slow, circular motion, lift your other arm out in front of you, then vertically up into the air. Let it gently continue the circle behind your body, and then complete the circle by letting it hang by your side where it started. Repeat this circular motion 8–10 times and then perform with the opposite arm.

1 2 3

4 5 6

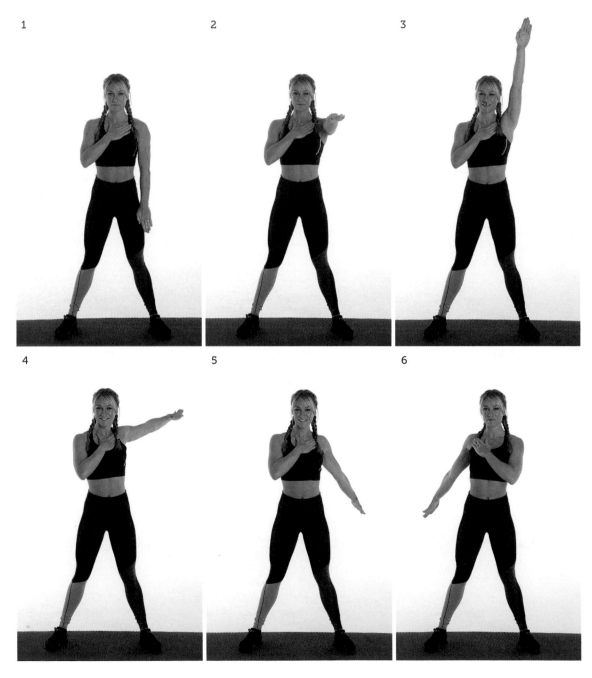

SHOULDER STRETCH

WARM UP & COOL DOWN
Stand up straight with your feet hip-width apart. Let your arms hang down by your sides. Lift one arm out in front of you. Reach your opposite hand across your body, under your armpit, and flatten your hand behind the extended arm's shoulder. Slowly and gently use your flattened hand to push against the back of the shoulder, extending the arm across your upper body, so it is horizontal across your chest. Repeat with the opposite arm.

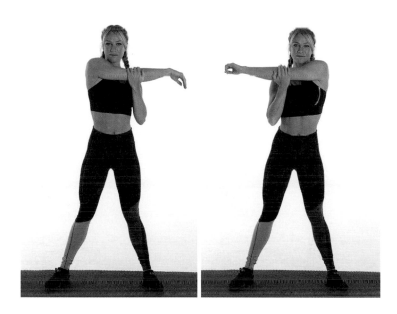

TRICEP STRETCH

WARM UP & COOL DOWN
Stand up straight with your feet hip-width apart. Lift one arm up into the air and then allow your forearm to hang down gently behind your head and neck. Using your opposite hand, gently grasp the back of your elbow/tricep area. Slowly push against this area so you feel a pull/stretch in your arm. Repeat with the opposite arm.

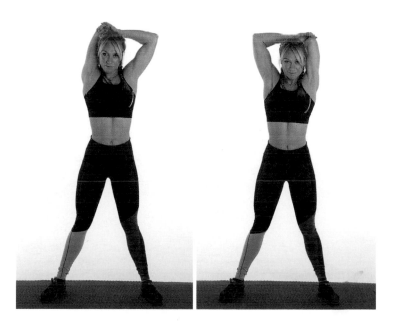

WRIST STRETCH

WARM UP ONLY Stand up straight with your feet hip-width apart. Extend both arms out to the sides (maintain a slight bend in your elbows). Slowly and gently roll your wrists outwards and inwards, in clockwise and anticlockwise movements respectively. Continue this movement for 8–10 seconds.

1

2

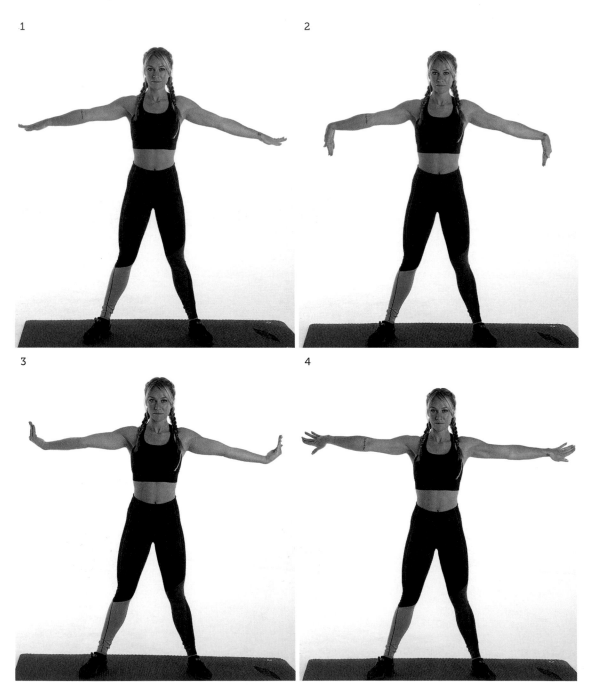

3

4

NECK STRETCH

WARM UP Stand up straight with your feet hip-width apart. Look straight ahead, then slowly and gently turn your head to one side, before coming back to centre. Then slowly and gently turn your head to the opposite side, before coming back to centre once again. Then look down, before coming back to centre, and finally look up, before coming back to centre again.

1   2   3

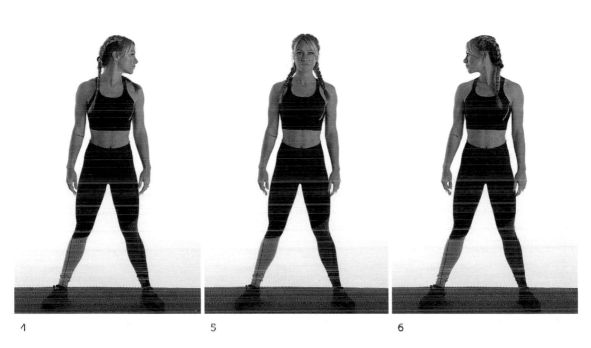

4   5   6

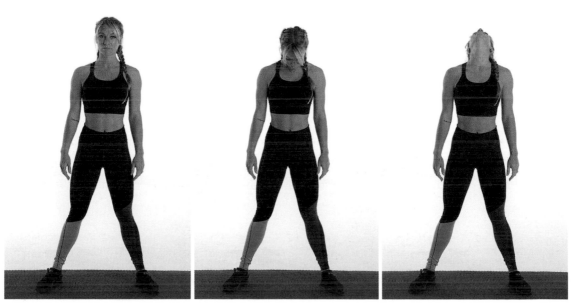

QUAD STRETCH

WARM UP & COOL DOWN
You may need to hold on to something to keep your balance while doing this. Stand up straight with your feet together. Bend one knee, lifting one foot up behind your body, and grasp the foot with your hand. Slowly and gently pull your foot upwards, so you feel a pull/stretch down the front of your leg/quad. Repeat with your opposite leg.

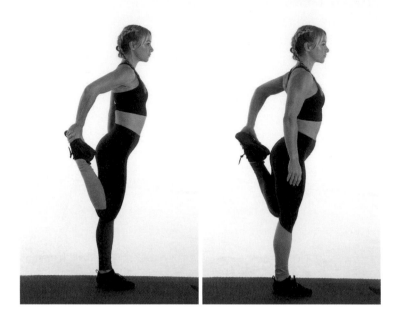

KNEE CIRCLES

WARM UP ONLY Stand with your feet together and bend down slightly so your hands fit in between your knees. Gently circle your knees in a clockwise direction 8 times, before repeating in the opposite direction.

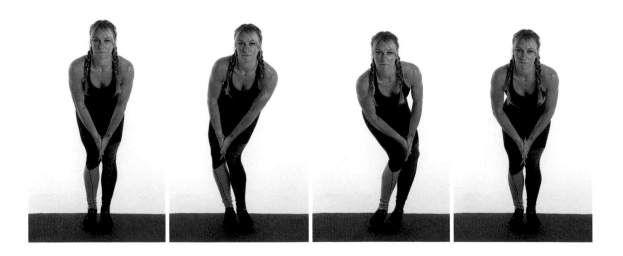

HAMSTRING STRETCH

WARM UP & COOL DOWN
Stand up straight with your feet together. Slowly and gently bend one knee (rest your hands on this knee to balance or, alternatively, place your hands on your hips). Slowly and gently stretch the opposite leg out in front of you, resting on the heel, toes pointing upwards. Keep your shoulders relaxed and feel the stretch in the back of your outstretched leg/hamstring. Repeat this movement with your opposite leg. Repeat with each leg 8–10 times to warm up. Hold each stretch for 8–10 seconds to cool down.

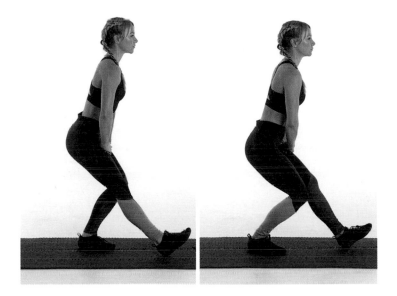

HIP OPENER

WARM UP & COOL DOWN Stand with your legs apart, toes facing outwards. Keeping your back straight at all times, slowly and gently come down into a low squat. Rest your elbows on your knees for balance. Slowly and gently lean to the right, stretching out your left hip. Repeat on each side 8–10 times to warm up. Hold each stretch for 8–10 seconds to cool down.

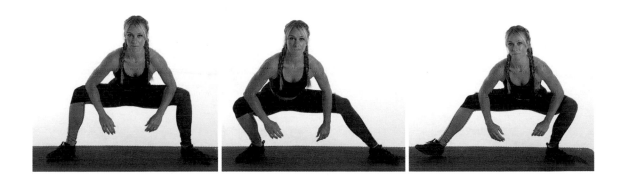

GLUTE STRETCH

WARM UP & COOL DOWN
Stand on your left leg and place your right ankle on top of your left thigh. Lower yourself down into a seated position – you will feel the stretch in the right side of your glute (buttocks). You can help the stretch by pressing gently on top of your right knee. Repeat with the opposite leg. If you have trouble keeping your balance, you can find something to hold on to.

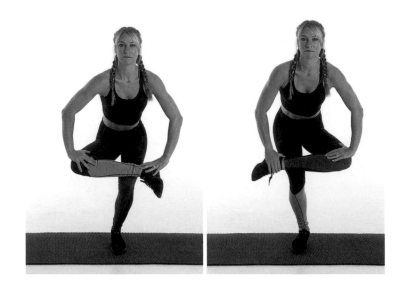

CALF STRETCH

WARM UP & COOL DOWN
Stand up straight with your feet together. Place your hands on your hips and lunge forward on one leg, as far as you can within your natural range. Keeping your back leg straight, try and push your back heel down to the ground – you should feel a stretch/pull in your calf muscle. Repeat with the opposite leg.

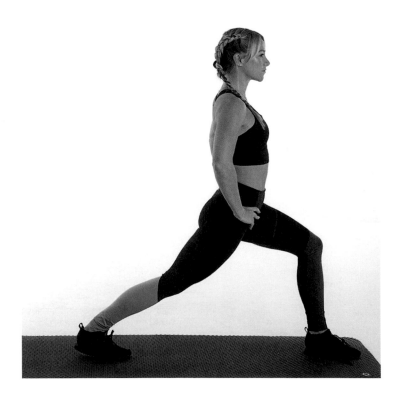

CHEST/BACK STRETCH

WARM UP ONLY Stand up straight with your feet hip-width apart. Raise your arms up to chest height and slowly and gently try to touch your elbows behind your back, within your natural range. Slowly and gently bring your arms back in front of your chest and cross your arms, almost like you are giving yourself a hug. Repeat this movement 8–10 times.

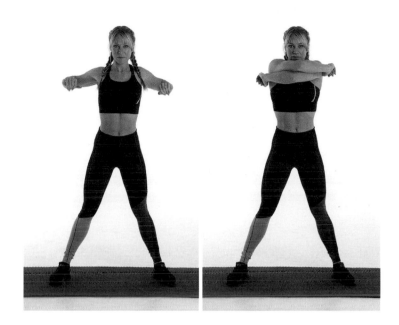

CHEST/BACK STRETCH

WARM UP & COOL DOWN Stand up straight with your feet hip-width apart. Let your arms hang loose at your sides before gently holding your hands behind your back. Slowly and gently extend your arms behind you, within your natural range, and try to pull your shoulders back and push your chest out.

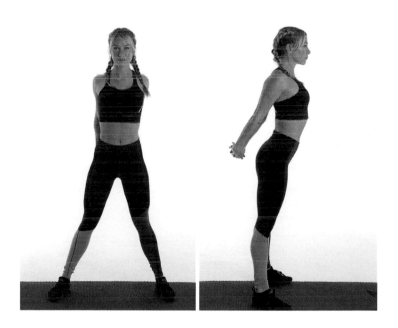

ANKLE ROLLS

WARM UP ONLY Using
a simple circular motion,
rotate each foot at the
ankle for 10 circuits in
each direction.

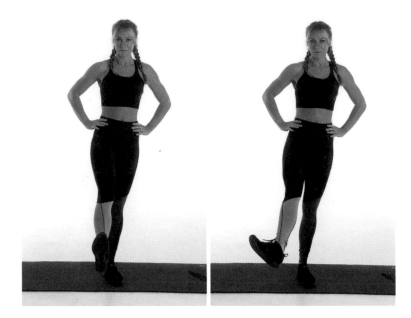

AB STRETCH

WARM UP & COOL DOWN
Stand up straight with your
feet hip-width apart. Raise
your arms up above your
head and lace your fingers
together, palms facing the
ceiling. Extend your upper
body upwards as much as
you can within your range.
You should feel a stretch up
the front of your torso and
also up the back of your
spine. After holding this
position for 8–10 seconds,
keep your back straight and
slowly and gently bend to
one side. You will feel a pull
along the side of your torso.
Repeat on the opposite side.

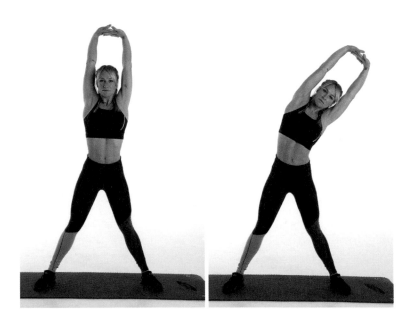

BACK STRETCH

WARM UP & COOL DOWN
Stand up straight with your feet hip-width apart. Crossing your arms in front of you, let them wrap all the way around your chest, like you are giving yourself a hug. With your hands flat against the backs of your shoulders, perform a gentle pull – you should feel this stretch in the centre of your back. Slowly bend down, creating a convex shape with your spine.

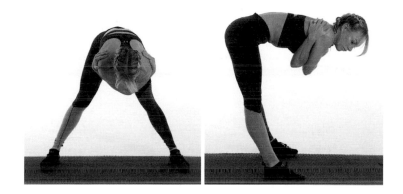

BICEP STRETCH

WARM UP & COOL DOWN
Stand up straight with your feet hip-width apart. Extend one arm out in front of you, your fingertips pointing upwards, your palm facing forwards. Place your opposite arm slightly above the other, your fingertips facing downwards, your palm facing inwards. Slide this hand over the other and slowly and gently pull. You will feel a stretch along the inside of your arm. Repeat with the opposite arm.

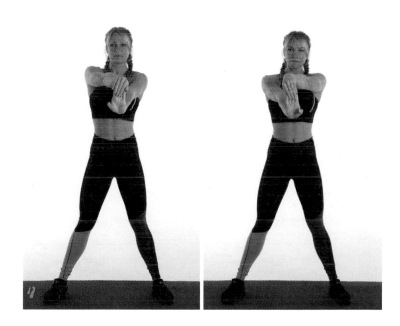

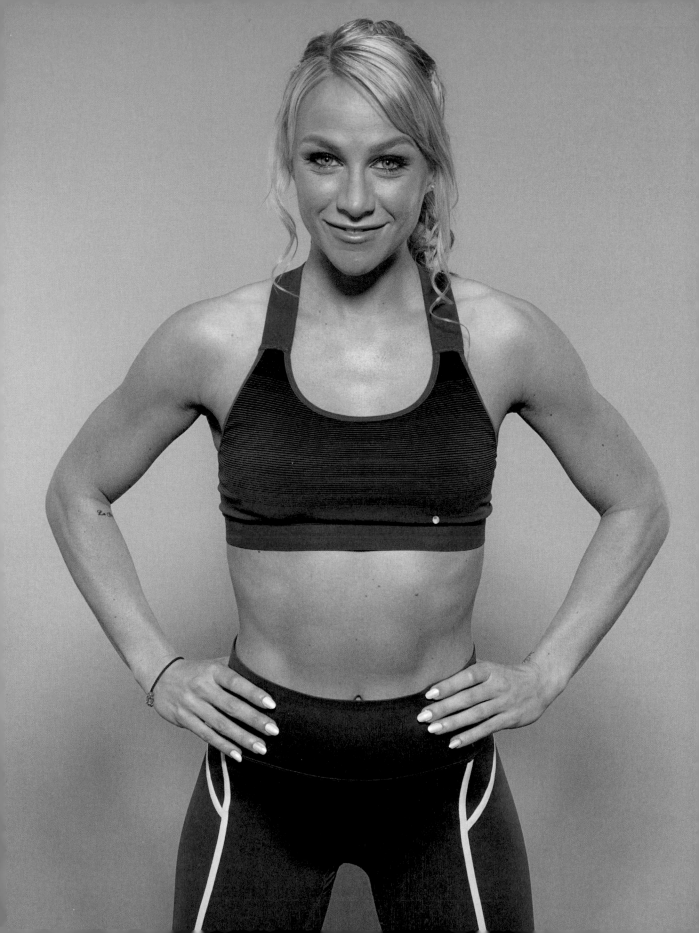

THE
SEDENTARY
PLAN

THE SEDENTARY DIET PLAN

Your diet will not change or progress during the 4 weeks of this plan. This is because I want to slowly and gradually increase your energy *output* (exercise), instead of slowly and gradually decreasing your energy *input* (food).

While you do need to change *one* of the above to continue to progress, I would *much* rather change your *output* than your *input*.

This is because if you are sedentary/unfit/out of shape/in recovery then your fitness levels need to progress gradually while your nutritional health remains well balanced.

Your DAILY food intake will look like this:

1. Breakfast
2. Snack
3. Lunch
4. Snack
5. Dinner

» You can eat these in any order/combination but you must eat *every single* meal and snack *daily*.

» Sedentary Plan followers should make sure to eat *before* any exercise and *after* any exercise.

Use the tables on pages 23–31 to build your own meals, or go to pages 152–213 for my recipes.

1. BREAKFAST
CHOOSE
1 protein option
1 carbohydrate option
1 veg option
OR
1 high-carb breakfast recipe

2. SNACK*
1 protein option
*Men to replace with 1 **high**-carb meal*

3. LUNCH
CHOOSE
1 protein option
1 carbohydrate option
1 veg option
OR
1 high-carb lunch or dinner recipe

4. SNACK*
1 protein option
*Men to replace with 1 **low**-carb meal*

5. DINNER
CHOOSE
1 protein option
1 fat option
1 veg option
OR
1 low-carb lunch or dinner recipe

♂ Men must replace both daily snack options with meals to ensure they hit an appropriate calorie count.

TELL ME WHY...

I have calculated your daily calorie and macronutrient intakes to get you results *without* you having to do anything too advanced, like implement a carb cycle (intermittent high-carb and low-carb days throughout the week).

There *are* plans in this book where I do instruct a carb cycle, but it is *totally* unnecessary for a complete beginner and, without the right training in place, it is not as effective as it could and/or should be.

Let me be very clear right now...
Carbs at night do not make you fat

I repeat...
Carbs at night do not make you fat!

So why have I replaced your breakfast and lunch carbs for fats at dinner?

❯❯ Simply because eating carbs earlier in the day will help your blood sugar and brain energy levels.

❯❯ Consuming fats later in the day helps to ensure you get this pivotal macronutrient in your daily diet. Keeping carbs and fats separate in your daily meals also helps you keep your calories in check during the day.

Remember...
IF YOU WANT THE RESULTS
YOU HAVE TO STICK TO THE DIET!
You will not get what you want out of this plan
if you have an extra snack here and a late night
pizza there. For the next few weeks, you need
to be committed to your physical health.
Take care of your body – feed it well,
train it well, rest it well and you will
get the results you want.

THE SEDENTARY TRAINING PLAN

What I am about to tell you is not mind-blowing – I have not reinvented the wheel – but it is true to say that if you are sedentary, unfit and/or out of shape, you need to start from square one and gradually work your way up to general strength and fitness.

My training plan for you is an easy, tried-and-tested way to do that.

However, no matter how rudimental this plan may seem, believe me when I tell you that if you execute this diet and training plan 100%, you absolutely *will* see aesthetic results in a matter of weeks.

The fact of the matter is you will be exerting more energy via exercise and intaking less energy via food. You will be in a calorie deficit and you will be physically active, this is an inevitable fat-loss formula.

Once you've completed your progressive 4-week plan, you can no longer call yourself a fitness beginner. However, if you want to stay on this plan you can – for up to 24 weeks in total.

While I want you to stick to the exercise plan *most* days of the week, if you'd like to replace the odd session every few days with:

>> Swimming
>> A gym class
>> A PT session
>> Any cardio machine you like
>> Any sporting activity (weekly training/games)

that is totally fine...

As long as you stick to the minimum times and days instructed!

Feel free to exercise at any time of day, whenever suits you best. However, don't forget that you must exercise *after* you've eaten one of your meals or snacks, and *before* another meal or snack.

Any day without training is a day of rest.

TELL ME WHY...

You will notice that you begin with low to moderate intensity cardio *only*, which is not only *appropriate* for beginners, but also *effective* for beginners.

I don't care *what* kind of cardio you choose to do (walking/cross trainer/swimming/gym class/PT session etc.) as long as you stick to the minimum times and days instructed each week.

Over the course of the following week, I want you to try to increase this low to moderate intensity whenever and wherever possible. In week 2, you should attempt intermittent jogging (if you are using a cardio machine, simply up the speed; if you are swimming simply increase your speed or change the difficulty of the stroke). This is to ensure that *not only* do we continue to increase your fitness levels, but we continue to increase your overall aesthetic progress as well.

The final 2 weeks see you doing resistance training (using muscle) in the first half of a circuit. The second half of the circuit sees your first HIIT session (high intensity interval training).

Now, I know you will be only 2 weeks into exercising at this point, but from previous clients and experience, I am confident that a short burst of HIIT will be manageable. However, if you struggle, take it nice and slow and just try to keep moving from beginning to end.

You will also notice that in the final 2 weeks, your circuit and low to moderate intensity cardio days are broken up. This is because intense training can cause stress to the body and inflammation to boot. Adding in low to moderate intensity cardio in place of resistance and HIIT on intermittent days is going to help your body recover, respond and make the changes we're aiming for.

WEEK 1

LOW–MODERATE INTENSITY CARDIO x 30 MINUTES

FAST-PACED WALKING (UPHILL IF / WHEN / WHERE POSSIBLE) OR ANY CARDIO MACHINE (SLIGHT RESISTANCE) OR SWIMMING OR GYM CLASS OR PT SESSION

ON ANY 5 DAYS OF THE WEEK

WEEK 1 TOTAL: 2½ HOURS

WEEK 2

LOW–MODERATE INTENSITY CARDIO x 40 MINUTES

FAST-PACED WALKING (UPHILL IF / WHEN / WHERE POSSIBLE) INTERSPERSED WITH INTERMITTENT JOGGING OR ANY CARDIO MACHINE (SLIGHT RESISTANCE) OR SWIMMING OR GYM CLASS OR PT SESSION

ON ANY 6 DAYS OF THE WEEK

WEEK 2 TOTAL: 4 HOURS

Monday + Wednesday + Friday

WARM UP (SEE PAGES 42–51)

CIRCUIT (SEE PAGES 60–62)
EXERCISES 1–4: 1 MINUTE EACH » REST: 1 MINUTE
REPEAT x 5 TIMES
TOTAL: 25 MINUTES

+

HIIT CARDIO (SEE PAGE 63)
BURPEES: $\frac{1}{2}$ MINUTE » REST: $1\frac{1}{2}$ MINUTES
REPEAT x 10 TIMES » **100% EFFORT!**
TOTAL: 20 MINUTES

COOL DOWN (SEE PAGES 42–51)

TOTAL: 45 MINUTES

Tuesday + Thursday + Saturday

LOW–MODERATE INTENSITY CARDIO
FAST-PACED WALKING (UPHILL IF/WHEN/WHERE POSSIBLE)
OR ANY CARDIO MACHINE (SLIGHT RESISTANCE)
OR SWIMMING

45 MINUTES PER DAY

CIRCUIT MONDAY + WEDNESDAY + FRIDAY

1 STANDING SQUATS x 1 minute

Stand up straight with your feet hip-width apart. Extend your arms directly out in front of you and place one hand on top of the other – alternatively, place your hands on your hips. Keeping your back straight, lower yourself down into a deep squat by bending your hips, then knees. Pushing your weight down against your heels, stand back up straight again. Make sure your knees stay directly above your toes – they shouldn't be collapsing inward. Repeat this movement for 1 minute.

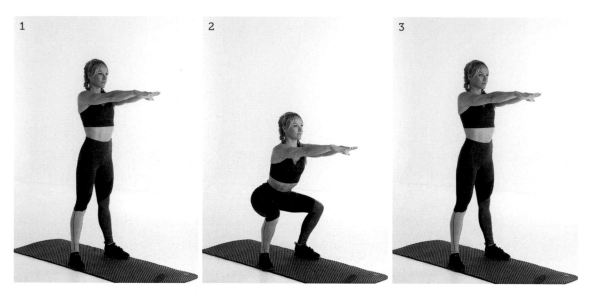

2 HIP THRUSTS x 1 minute

You may need a mat or a soft surface for this exercise. Lie on your back with your feet hip-width apart and your knees bent. Slowly and gently raise your hips up into the air, squeezing your buttocks as you do so. Hold this position for a few seconds before slowly and gently coming back down to your starting position. Repeat this movement for 1 minute.

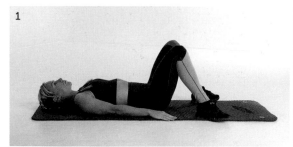
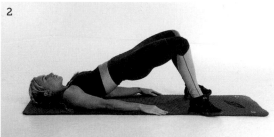

3 THE PLANK x 1 minute

You may need a mat or cushion for your elbows during this exercise. Lie on your front with your feet hip-width apart, resting your toes against the top of the mat. Rest on your elbows and keep your forearms flat against the mat. Make sure your elbows are below your shoulders. Pushing against your toes and forearms, raise your body up into the air to form an elevated plank. DO NOT allow your spine to curve, either concavely or convexly. You want a straight back. Try to hold this position for 1 minute. If you are struggling, feel free to transfer your weight from one foot to another, essentially shuffling your feet while holding the plank position. Alternatively, come back down on to the mat for a couple of seconds to catch your breath and then return to the plank position to complete the minute.

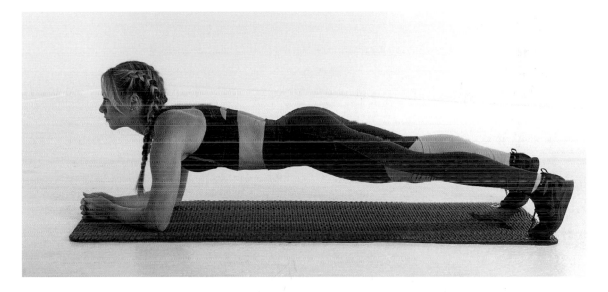

These circuits separate your resistance exercises and HIIT cardio intentionally. I want you to focus on contracting your muscles during your circuit and then focus on giving 100% effort to your HIIT.

4 WALK OUT PUSH UPS x 1 minute

Stand up straight with your feet hip-width apart. Allowing your knees to bend slightly, come down and forwards, so that your hands touch the floor, palms flat, and shoulder-width apart. Crawl forwards until you are fully extended in a horizontal position. Keeping your back straight and bending only at the elbows, perform a push up. Crawl your hands back until you can stand upright again. Repeat this movement for 1 minute.

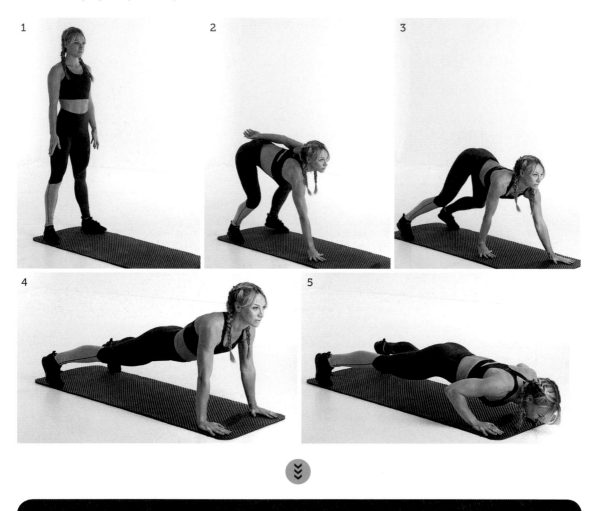

REST: 1 MINUTE
REPEAT EXERCISES 1–4 AND REST x 5 TIMES
TOTAL: 25 MINUTES

HIIT MONDAY + WEDNESDAY + FRIDAY

HIIT CARDIO
BURPEES: ½ MINUTE » REST: 1½ MINUTES
REPEAT x 10 TIMES » 100% EFFORT!
TOTAL: 20 MINUTES

HIIT » BURPEES
100% EFFORT!

Stand up straight with your feet together and your arms down by your sides. »» Come down into a crouch and place your palms flat on the ground in front of you. »» Put your body weight on your hands and jump your legs backwards, so you are in a plank position but resting on your hands, not on your elbows. »» Jump your legs back in, knees to your chest, to return to your crouch position. »» Finally, explode up into the air in a jump, landing back in your starting position. »» Continue this movement for ½ minute at 100% effort, then rest for 1½ minutes. Repeat 10 times.

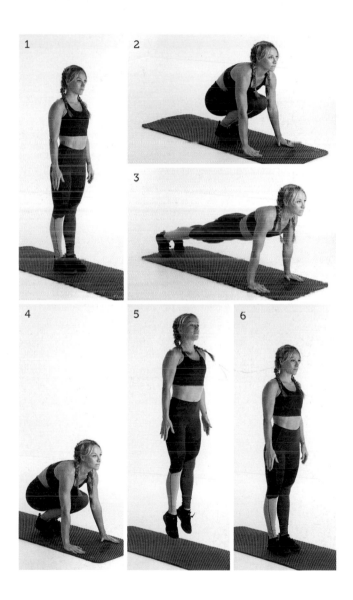

Monday + Wednesday + Friday

WARM UP (SEE PAGES 42–51)

CIRCUIT (SEE PAGES 65–66)
EXERCISES 1–4: 1 MINUTE EACH » REST: 1 MINUTE
REPEAT x 5 TIMES
TOTAL: 25 MINUTES

+

HIIT CARDIO (SEE PAGE 67)
MOUNTAIN CLIMBERS: $\frac{1}{2}$ MINUTE »
REST: $1\frac{1}{2}$ MINUTES
REPEAT x 11 TIMES » **100% EFFORT!**
TOTAL: 22 MINUTES

COOL DOWN (SEE PAGES 42–51)

Tuesday + Thursday + Saturday

LOW-MODERATE INTENSITY CARDIO
FAST-PACED WALKING (UPHILL IF/WHEN/WHERE POSSIBLE)
OR ANY CARDIO MACHINE (SLIGHT RESISTANCE)
OR SWIMMING
45 MINUTES PER DAY

CIRCUIT MONDAY + WEDNESDAY + FRIDAY

1 ALTERNATE LUNGES x 1 minute

Stand up straight with your feet together and your hands on your hips. Lunge forward with one leg, as far as your natural range will allow. Bending your knees, push down into the lunge, allowing your back knee to hover just above floor level and keeping your front knee directly above your toes. Push back up into your starting position and repeat with the opposite leg. Perform alternately for 1 minute.

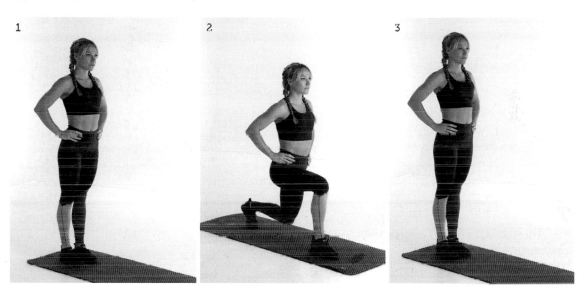

2 GLUTE BRIDGE HOLD x 1 minute

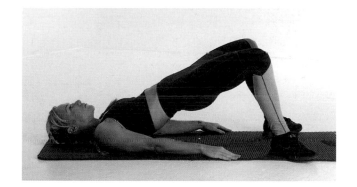

This is similar to a Hip Thrust but *without* the repetitive movement... You may need a mat or a soft surface for this exercise. Lie on your back with your feet hip-width apart and your knees bent. Slowly and gently thrust your hips up into the air, squeezing your buttocks as you do so. Hold this position at the peak of the thrust and continue to squeeze your buttocks. Hold this move for 1 minute.

3 ELBOWS TO HAND PLANK x 1 minute

You may need a mat or cushion for your elbows during this exercise. Lie on your front with your feet hip-width apart, resting your toes against the top of the mat. Lean on your elbows and keep your forearms flat against the mat. Make sure your elbows are below your shoulders. Pushing against your toes and forearms, raise your upper body into the air, one arm at a time, to rest on your hands, so you form an elevated plank. DO NOT allow your spine to curve, either concavely or convexly. You want a straight back. Come back down to rest on your forearms, one arm at a time, and then push back up on to your hands. Repeat this movement for 1 minute.

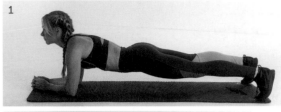

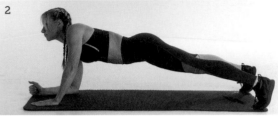

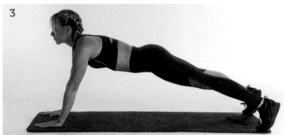

4 PUSH UPS x 1 minute

Stand up straight with your feet hip-width apart. Allowing your knees to bend slightly, come down and forwards, allowing your hands to touch the floor, palms flat and shoulder-width apart. Crawl outwards until you are fully extended in a horizontal position. Keeping your back straight and bending only at the elbows, perform a push up. Repeat this move for 1 minute. If you need to come on to your knees to complete the full minute, you may do so.

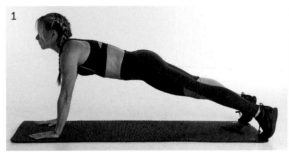

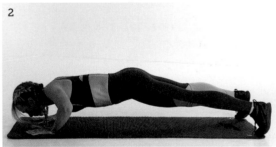

REST: 1 MINUTE
REPEAT EXERCISES 1–4 AND REST x 5 TIMES
TOTAL: 25 MINUTES

HIIT CARDIO
MOUNTAIN CLIMBERS: ½ MINUTE » REST: 1½ MINUTES
REPEAT x 11 TIMES » 100% EFFORT!
TOTAL: 22 MINUTES

HIIT »
MOUNTAIN CLIMBERS
100% EFFORT!

Lie on your front, feet hip-width apart, toes on the floor. » Place your hands by the sides of your chest, palms to the floor. » Push yourself up using your hands and feet. » Bring one knee up to your chest and then return it to the starting position. As you do this, switch legs. » Continue this movement for ⅓ minute at 100% effort then rest for 1½ minutes. Repeat 11 times.

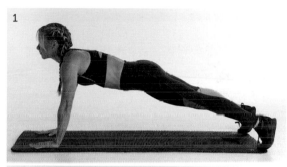

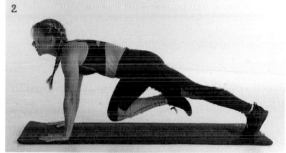

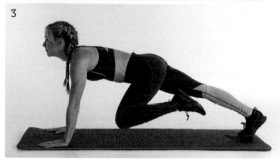

HIIT is hard but its metabolic effects are incredible. The more oomph you give it, the more beneficial it is!

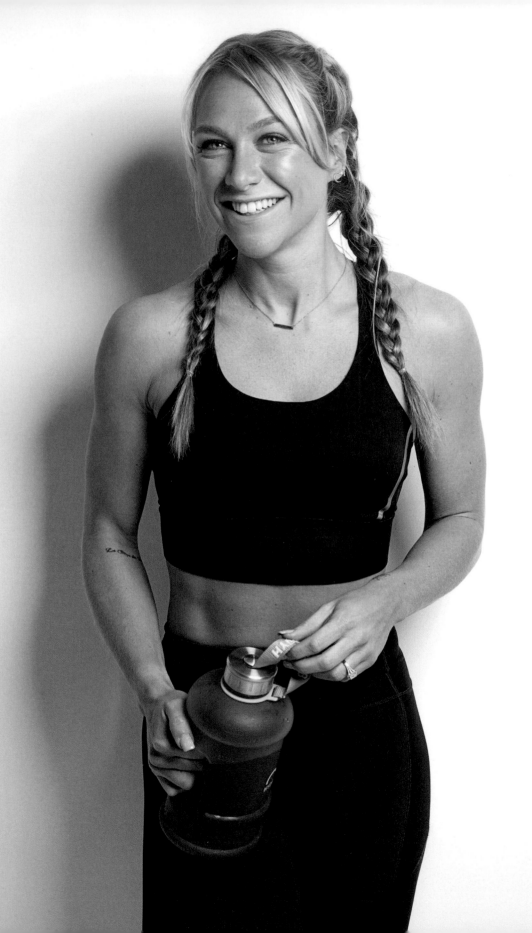

THE
ACTIVE
PLAN

THE ACTIVE DIET PLAN

For this plan I am giving you a WEEKLY carb cycle, structured as follows:

›› 5 days low calorie via low carb (depletion)

›› 2 days higher calorie via high carb (re-feed)

Your WEEKLY food intake will look like this:

Monday – Low-carb Meals and Snacks

Tuesday – Low-carb Meals and Snacks

Wednesday – Low-carb Meals and Snacks

Thursday – Low-carb Meals and Snacks

Friday – Low-carb Meals and Snacks

Saturday – High-carb Meals and Snacks (+1 extra carbohydrate snack)

Sunday – High-carb Meals and Snacks (+1 extra carbohydrate snack)

Your MONDAY – FRIDAY 5-day daily deficit intake will be as follows:

1. Breakfast
2. Snack
3. Lunch
4. Snack
5. Dinner

Your SATURDAY + SUNDAY 2-day re-feed intake will be as follows:

1. Breakfast
2. Snack
3. Lunch
4. Snack
5. Dinner
+
1 carbohydrate snack

›› You can eat these in any order/ combination, but you must eat *every single* meal and snack *daily*.

›› I also want you to make sure you *always* eat one of the above *after* any exercise.

Use the tables on pages 23–31 to build your own meals, or go to pages 159–213 for my recipes.

Monday – Friday
5-day daily deficit intake

1. BREAKFAST
CHOOSE
1 protein option
1 fat option
1 veg option
OR
1 low-carb breakfast recipe

2. SNACK*
1 protein option
*Men to replace with 1 **low**-carb meal*

3. LUNCH
CHOOSE
1 protein option
1 fat option
1 veg option
OR
1 low-carb lunch or dinner recipe

4. SNACK*
1 protein option
*Men to replace with 1 **low**-carb meal*

5. DINNER
CHOOSE
1 protein option
1 fat option
1 veg option
OR
1 low-carb lunch or dinner recipe

♂ Men must replace both daily snack options with **low-carb** meal options to ensure they hit an appropriate caloric count.

Saturday + Sunday
2-day re-feed intake

1. BREAKFAST
CHOOSE
1 protein option
1 carb option
1 veg option
OR
1 high-carb breakfast recipe

2. SNACK*
1 protein option
*Men to replace with 1 **high**-carb meal*

3. LUNCH
CHOOSE
1 protein option
1 carb option
1 veg option
OR
1 high-carb lunch or dinner recipe

4. SNACK*
1 protein option
*Men to replace with 1 **high**-carb meal*

5. DINNER
CHOOSE
1 protein option
1 carb option
1 veg option
OR
1 high-carb lunch or dinner recipe

6. SNACK*
1 carbohydrate snack
*Men to replace with 1 **high**-carb meal*

♂ Men must replace all three daily snack options with **high-carb** meal options to ensure they hit an appropriate calorie count.

TELL ME WHY...

The reasons I am implementing a 5/2 SPLIT are as follows:

>> 5 days in a calorie deficit (via carb depletion) will inevitably lead to a loss.

>> Implementing two consecutive weekly re-feeds (via carb increases) will feed your muscle, allowing you to refuel, recover and continue to train hard over the course of the next few days:

> The first re-feed will *halt* the drastic drop in hormonal and metabolic functions that are inevitable when implementing a low-calorie, fat-loss phase. This drop in hormonal and metabolic function is what leads to the infamous plateau.

> The second re-feed will ramp your hormonal and metabolic levels back up, allowing you to re-enter your depletion and continue to lose effectively, week on week, until you are ready to end *The Fat-Loss Blitz*.

Additional Benefits of the 5/2 SPLIT:

>> A lot of my Blitzers take part in group sports and teams tend to play at the weekends. These weekend re-feeds are a great way to go out there fully fuelled for a game and recover in the hours after.

>> Most of us have social events at the weekends. While you are not permitted to 'cheat' or drink alcohol on *The Fat-Loss Blitz*, having two higher calorie and carb days can make going out for meals a little less intimidating.

THE ACTIVE TRAINING PLAN

Let me start by saying that, although the Active Plan is similar to *The 4-Week Body Blitz*, it also has some pretty notable differences.

What I have learned from my Blitzers is that you guys *thrive* when given the freedom to be active in whichever way you please – be this a gym class, a weekly game of rugby or netball, a PT session or an outdoor run.

While I *do* want you to stick to my exercise plan *most* days of the week, if you would like to replace the odd session with:

>> Swimming

>> A gym class

>> A PT session

>> Any cardio machine you like

>> Any sporting activity
   (weekly training/games)

that is totally fine...

As long as you stick to the minimum times and days instructed!

This plan requires you to train 6 days a week. This is because of the varying training intensities and weekly re-feed days. However, if you *need* to implement an added rest day, you may do so.

If you *do* choose to do this, I suggest you make it as close to your first re-feed day as possible, as this is when your body will likely need rest most and will recover best.

Any day without training is a day of rest.

TELL ME WHY...

Your circuits have been broken up into two parts:

1. Resistance

2. HIIT (high intensity interval training)

I want you to be able to focus 100% on *feeling* the contraction of muscle as you perform each exercise. This is because mind to muscle connection is a very good way to ensure that you get the best results and muscular development from your resistance training.

Equally, when it comes to your HIIT, I want you to be able to focus on giving it **100% all-out effort**, instead of feeling fatigued from the overall circuit.

By splitting resistance and HIIT up in this way, I am hoping you get even better aesthetic results.

You will also notice that I have *not* instructed you to perform HIIT 5–6 times weekly like I did in my last book. Instead, your HIIT and low-moderate intensity cardio days are now broken up.

This is because intense training can cause stress to the body and inflammation to boot. Adding in low to moderate intensity cardio in place of HIIT on intermittent days is going to help your body recover, respond and make the changes we're aiming for.

Don't panic over the loss of daily HIIT, *all* cardio is effective and they *all* trump each other in one way or another.

For example, while HIIT is a great metabolic booster, doing it *too* often can have the *reverse* effect, and can slow down results owing to stress on the body.

Low-intensity cardio can alleviate said stress and encourage your body to recover and respond again.

Moderate intensity cardio is a great way to encourage a fat-burning state specifically.

So, as I say, *all* cardio is effective in some way and you should implement every style for optimum aesthetic results.

THE ACTIVE TRAINING PLAN

Monday – Saturday
WARM UP (SEE PAGES 42–51)
RESISTANCE CIRCUIT
EXERCISES 1–4: 1 MINUTE EACH » REST: 1 MINUTE
REPEAT x 5 TIMES
TOTAL: 25 MINUTES

FOLLOWED BY

Monday + Wednesday + Friday
HIIT CARDIO (SEE PAGE 79)
BURPEES: ½ MINUTE » REST: 1½ MINUTES
REPEAT x 10 TIMES » **100% EFFORT!**
TOTAL: 20 MINUTES

COOL DOWN (SEE PAGES 42–51)

OR

Tuesday + Thursday + Saturday
LOW–MODERATE INTENSITY CARDIO
FAST-PACED WALKING (UPHILL IF/WHEN/WHERE POSSIBLE)
OR ANY CARDIO MACHINE (SLIGHT RESISTANCE)
OR SWIMMING
20 MINUTES PER DAY

COOL DOWN (SEE PAGES 42–51)

1 STANDING SQUATS x 1 minute

Stand up straight with your feet hip-width apart. Extend your arms directly out in front of you and place one hand on top of the other – alternatively, place your hands on your hips. Keeping your back straight, lower yourself down into a deep squat by bending your hips, then knees. Pushing your weight down against your heels, stand back up straight again. Make sure your knees stay directly above your toes – they shouldn't be collapsing inward. Repeat this movement for 1 minute.

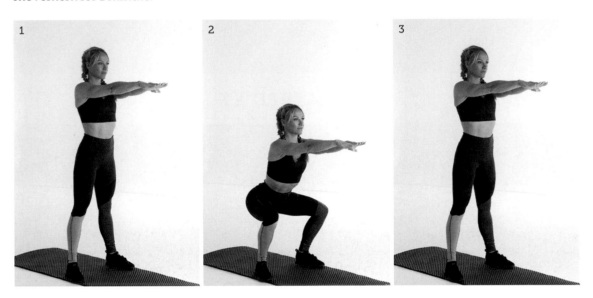

2 HIP THRUSTS x 1 minute

You may need a mat or a soft surface for this exercise. Lie on your back with your feet hip-width apart and your knees bent. Slowly and gently raise your hips up into the air, squeezing your buttocks as you do so. Hold this position for a few seconds before slowly and gently coming back down to your starting position. Repeat this movement for 1 minute.

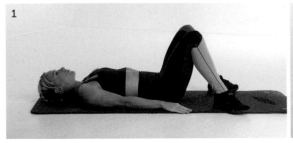
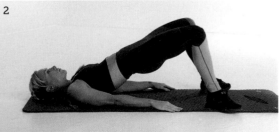

3 THE PLANK x 1 minute

You may need a mat or cushion for your elbows during this exercise. Lie on your front with your feet hip-width apart, resting your toes against the top of the mat. Rest on your elbows and keep your forearms flat against the mat. Make sure your elbows are below your shoulders. Pushing against your toes and forearms, raise your body up into the air to form an elevated plank. DO NOT allow your spine to curve, either concavely or convexly. You want a straight back. Try to hold this position for 1 minute. If you are struggling, feel free to transfer your weight from one foot to another, essentially shuffling your feet while holding the plank position. Alternatively, come back down on to the mat for a couple of seconds to catch your breath and then return to the plank position to complete the minute.

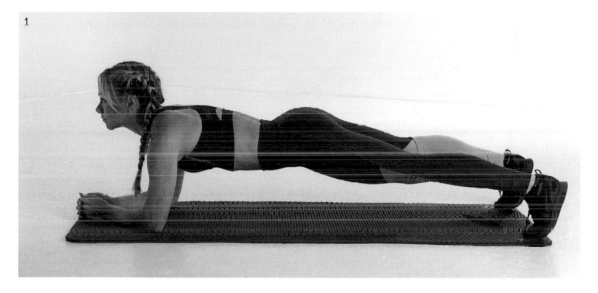

I want you to really focus on your
muscle during these circuits.
Engage the muscle that is supposed to
be working, and make sure you continue
to work it for the full minute.

CIRCUIT MONDAY – SATURDAY

4 WALK OUT PUSH UPS x 1 minute

Stand up straight with your feet hip-width apart. Allowing your knees to bend slightly, come down and forwards, so that your hands touch the floor, palms flat and shoulder-width apart. Crawl forwards until you are fully extended in a horizontal position. Keeping your back straight and bending only at the elbows, perform a push up. Crawl your hands back until you can stand upright again. Repeat this movement for 1 minute.

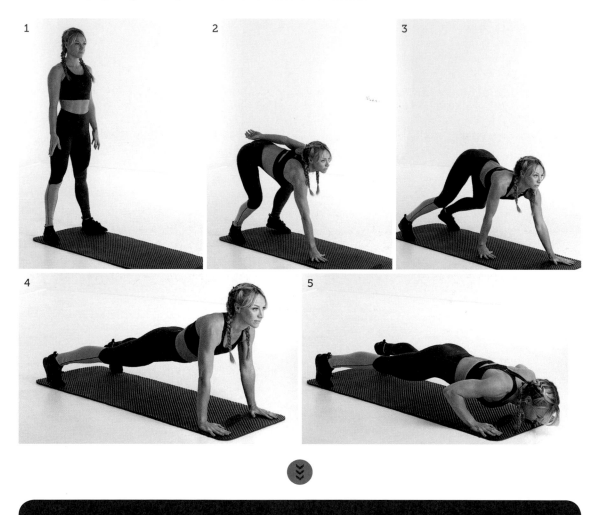

REST: 1 MINUTE
REPEAT EXERCISES 1–4 AND REST x 5 TIMES
TOTAL: 25 MINUTES

> ## HIIT CARDIO
> BURPEES: ½ MINUTE » REST: 1½ MINUTES
> REPEAT x 10 TIMES » 100% EFFORT!
> ## TOTAL: 20 MINUTES

HIIT » BURPEES
100% EFFORT!

Stand up straight with your feet together and your arms down by your sides. »› Come down into a crouch and place your palms flat on the ground in front of you. »› Put your body weight on your hands and jump your legs backwards, so you are in a plank position but resting on your hands, not on your elbows. »› Jump your legs back in, knees to your chest, to return to your crouch position. »› Finally, explode up into the air in a jump, landing back in your starting position. »› Continue this movement for ½ minute at 100% effort, then rest for 1½ minutes. Repeat 10 times.

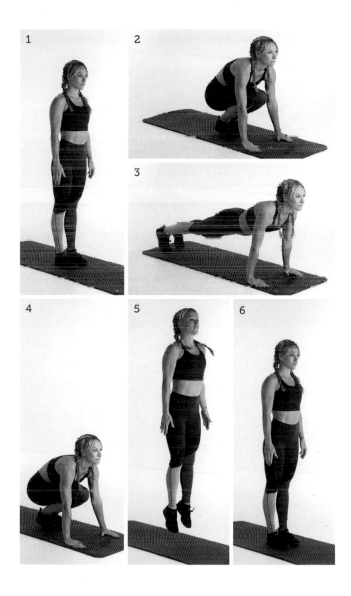

Monday – Saturday

WARM UP (SEE PAGES 42–51)

RESISTANCE CIRCUIT

EXERCISES 1–4: 1 MINUTE EACH » REST: 1 MINUTE
REPEAT x 5 TIMES
TOTAL: 25 MINUTES

FOLLOWED BY

Monday + Wednesday + Friday

HIIT CARDIO (SEE PAGE 83)

MOUNTAIN CLIMBERS: 1/2 MIN » REST: 1½ MINS
REPEAT x 11 TIMES » **100% EFFORT!**
TOTAL: 22 MINUTES

COOL DOWN (SEE PAGES 42–51)

OR

Tuesday + Thursday + Saturday

LOW–MODERATE INTENSITY CARDIO

FAST-PACED WALKING (UPHILL IF/WHEN/WHERE POSSIBLE)
OR ANY CARDIO MACHINE (SLIGHT RESISTANCE)
OR SWIMMING
25 MINUTES PER DAY

COOL DOWN (SEE PAGES 42–51)

CIRCUIT MONDAY – SATURDAY

1 ALTERNATE LUNGES x 1 minute

Stand up straight with your feet together and your hands on your hips. Lunge forward with one leg, as far as your natural range will allow. Bending your knees, push down into the lunge, allowing your back knee to hover just above floor level and keeping your front knee directly above your toes. Push back up into your starting position and repeat with the opposite leg. Perform alternately for 1 minute.

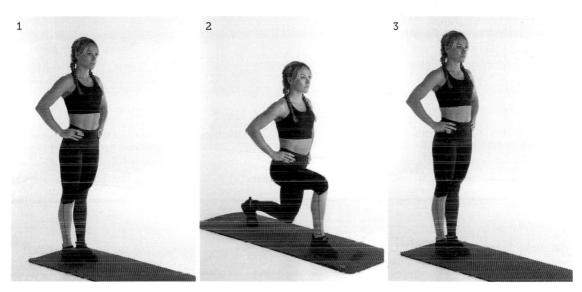

2 GLUTE BRIDGE HOLD x 1 minute

This is similar to a Hip Thrust but *without* the repetitive movement... You may need a mat or a soft surface for this exercise. Lie on your back with your feet hip-width apart and your knees bent. Slowly and gently thrust your hips up into the air, squeezing your buttocks as you do so. Hold this position at the peak of the thrust and continue to squeeze your buttocks. Hold this move for 1 minute.

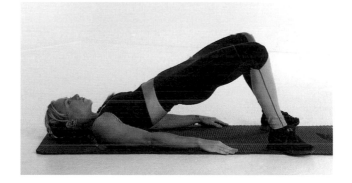

3 ELBOWS TO HAND PLANK x 1 minute

You may need a mat or cushion for your elbows during this exercise. Lie on your front with your feet hip-width apart, resting your toes against the top of the mat. Lean on your elbows and keep your forearms flat against the mat. Make sure your elbows are below your shoulders. Pushing against your toes and forearms, raise your upper body into the air, one arm at a time, to rest on your hands, so you form an elevated plank. DO NOT allow your spine to curve, either concavely or convexly. You want a straight back. Come back down to rest on your forearms, one arm at a time, and then push back up on to your hands. Repeat this movement for 1 minute.

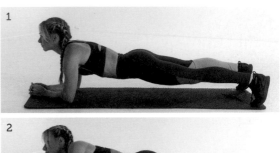

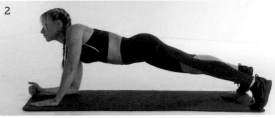

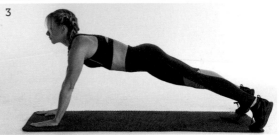

4 PUSH UPS x 1 minute

Stand up straight with your feet hip-width apart. Allowing your knees to bend slightly, come down and forwards, allowing your hands to touch the floor, palms flat and shoulder-width apart. Crawl outwards until you are fully extended in a horizontal position. Keeping your back straight and bending only at the elbows, perform a push up. Repeat this move for 1 minute. If you need to come on to your knees to complete the full minute, you may do so.

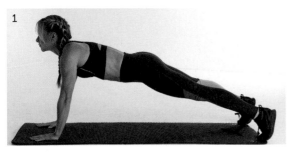

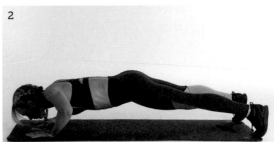

**REST: 1 MINUTE
REPEAT EXERCISES 1–4 AND REST x 5 TIMES
TOTAL: 25 MINUTES**

HIIT CARDIO
MOUNTAIN CLIMBERS: ½ MIN » REST: 1½ MINS
REPEAT × 11 TIMES » 100% EFFORT!
TOTAL: 22 MINUTES

HIIT »
MOUNTAIN CLIMBERS
100% EFFORT!

Lie on your front, feet hip-width apart, toes on the floor. » Place your hands by the sides of your chest, palms to the floor. » Push yourself up using your hands and feet. » Bring one knee up to your chest and then return it to the starting position. As you do this, switch legs. » Continue this movement for ½ minute at 100% effort then rest for 1½ minutes. Repeat 11 times.

I want you to give 100% effort for the full 30 seconds. The more effort you give, the better the effects of HIIT.

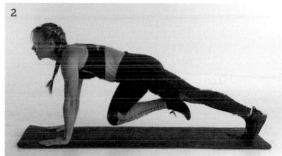

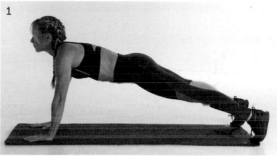

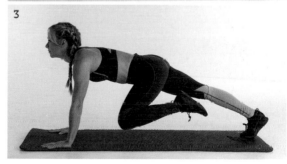

Monday – Saturday
WARM UP (SEE PAGES 42–51)
RESISTANCE CIRCUIT
EXERCISES 1–4: 1 MINUTE EACH » REST: 1 MINUTE
REPEAT x 5 TIMES
TOTAL: 25 MINUTES

FOLLOWED BY

Monday + Wednesday + Friday
HIIT CARDIO (SEE PAGE 87)
SQUAT JUMPS: $\frac{1}{2}$ MINUTE » REST: $1\frac{1}{2}$ MINUTES
REPEAT x 12 TIMES » **100% EFFORT!**
TOTAL: 24 MINUTES

COOL DOWN (SEE PAGES 42–51)

OR

Tuesday + Thursday + Saturday
LOW–MODERATE INTENSITY CARDIO
FAST-PACED WALKING (UPHILL IF/WHEN/WHERE POSSIBLE)
OR ANY CARDIO MACHINE (SLIGHT RESISTANCE)
OR SWIMMING
25 MINUTES PER DAY

COOL DOWN (SEE PAGES 42–51)

1 HEEL TAPS x 1 minute

You may need a mat or a soft surface to cushion your back for this exercise. Lie on your back with your knees bent and your feet flat on the floor and hip-width apart. Doing a very slight abdominal crunch so your upper back is slightly raised off the ground, stretch out your hands and move slowly to your right and left, repetitively, touching the outsides of your feet as you do so.

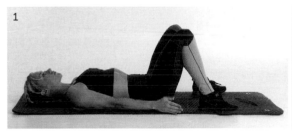

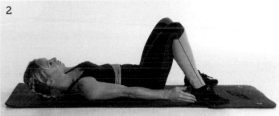

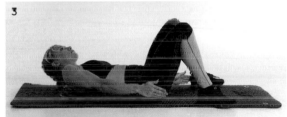

2 DONKEY SIDE KICKS x 1 minute

You may need a mat or a soft surface for this exercise. Get down on all fours. Make sure you keep your back straight – you don't want to do any damage by arching your spine during this exercise. Keeping the right-angle bend in your legs at all times, slowly raise one leg up and out to the side, until you feel the tension in your buttocks. Hold this position for 1 second before bringing your leg slowly back down to your starting position. Repeat with the opposite leg and continue to perform the exercise alternately for 1 minute.

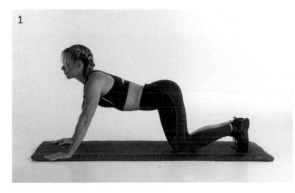

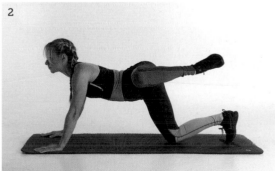

3 SIDE PLANK x 1 minute

You may need a mat or cushion for this exercise. Lie down on your side and prop your upper body up on your forearm (with a cushion underneath, if desired). Raise your outside hip up into the air and simultaneously push against your forearm and feet. Once one side of your body is raised in the air in a rigid, straight line, engage your core and hold this position for 30 seconds. Change sides and hold for another 30 seconds.

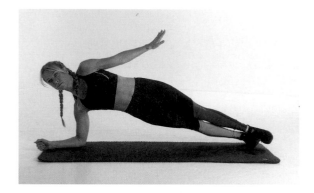

4 DIAMOND PUSH UPS x 1 minute

Stand up straight with your feet hip-width apart. Allowing your knees to bend slightly, come down and forwards, allowing your hands to touch the floor, palms flat, and thumbs and forefingers touching to form a diamond shape. Keeping your back straight and bending only at the elbows, perform a push up. Repeat this exercise for 1 minute. If you need to come on to your knees to complete the full minute, you may do so.

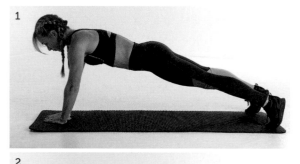

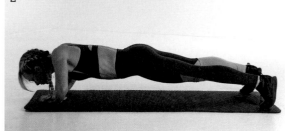

REST: 1 MINUTE
REPEAT EXERCISES 1–4 AND REST x 5 TIMES
TOTAL: 25 MINUTES

HIIT MONDAY + WEDNESDAY + FRIDAY

HIIT » SQUAT JUMPS 100% EFFORT!

Stand up straight with your feet hip-width apart. »» Extend your arms out in front of you and place one hand on top of the other – or place your hands on your hips, whichever is more comfortable. »» Keeping your back straight, lower yourself down into a deep squat by bending your knees. Instead of standing back up again from the squat, gently jump back into a standing position. The jump should be so gentle that you can maintain your form from the very start of the exercise to the next repetition. It should also be so gentle that you only come off the floor a little. Big dynamic jumps can damage your joints, so keep it gentle. »» Continue this movement for ½ minute at 100% effort then rest for 1½ minutes. Repeat 12 times.

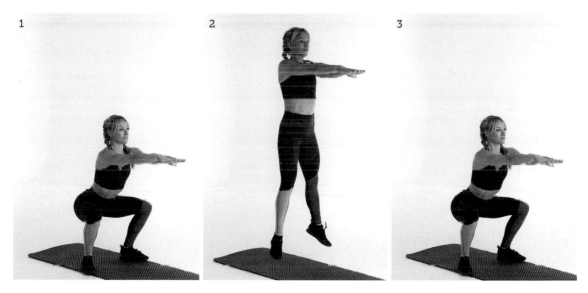

I find Squat Jumps harder than Burpees and
Mountain Climbers but everyone is different.
Really try to give 100% effort for the full 30 seconds
but if you need to slow it down a little, that's fine.

Monday – Saturday
WARM UP (SEE PAGES 42–51)
RESISTANCE CIRCUIT
EXERCISES 1–4: 1 MINUTE EACH » REST: 1 MINUTE
REPEAT x 5 TIMES
TOTAL: 25 MINUTES

FOLLOWED BY

Monday + Wednesday + Friday
HIIT CARDIO (SEE PAGE 91)
BURPEES: $\frac{1}{2}$ MINUTE » REST: $1\frac{1}{2}$ MINUTES
REPEAT x 13 TIMES » **100% EFFORT!**
TOTAL: 26 MINUTES

COOL DOWN (SEE PAGES 42–51)

OR

Tuesday + Thursday + Saturday
LOW–MODERATE INTENSITY CARDIO
FAST-PACED WALKING (UPHILL IF/WHEN/WHERE POSSIBLE)
OR ANY CARDIO MACHINE (SLIGHT RESISTANCE)
OR SWIMMING
30 MINUTES PER DAY

COOL DOWN (SEE PAGES 42–51)

CIRCUIT MONDAY – SATURDAY

1 SIDE LUNGES x 1 minute

Stand up straight with your feet together and your hands clasped in front of your chest. Take a big step out to one side with your left leg. Once you have planted your left foot on the floor, bend your right knee and come down into a side lunge. This will stretch out your left leg. Once you have come down as far as you can (within your natural range), push yourself back into your starting position. Repeat this movement with the opposite leg. Continue to perform alternately for 1 minute.

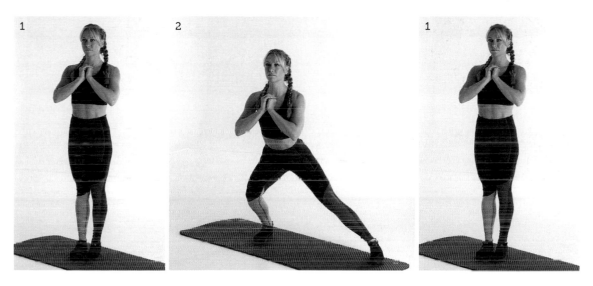

2 DONKEY KICK BACKS x 1 minute

You may need a mat or a soft surface for this exercise. Get down on all fours. Make sure to keep your back straight – you don't want to do any damage by arching your spine during this exercise. Keeping the right-angle bend in your legs at all times, slowly raise one leg up into the air behind you, as far as your natural range will allow, and then 'kick back' further. Hold this position for a second before slowly bringing your leg back down to your starting postition. Repeat the movement with the opposite leg and continue to perform alternately for 1 minute.

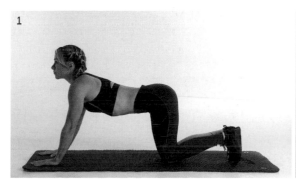
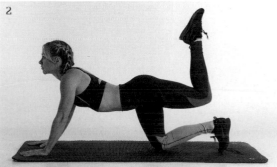

CIRCUIT MONDAY – SATURDAY

3 BICYCLES x 1 minute

You may need a mat or a soft surface for this exercise. Lie on your back and, keeping your knees and feet together, raise your lower body up off the ground so your legs are bent at a 90-degree angle. Place your hands up by the sides of your head, elbows bent and pointing towards your knees. Slowly come up into a slight abdominal crunch and move your right elbow to your left knee, followed by your left elbow to your right knee. Continue to perform this exercise fluidly for 1 minute.

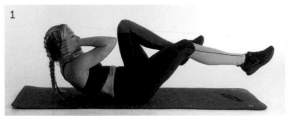
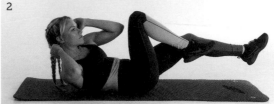

4 TRICEP DIPS x 1 minute

You will need a chair, a step, a bench, or any slightly raised surface for this exercise. Stand facing away from the chair but place your hands behind you, palms flat down on the chair. Lower your body slowly by bending at the elbows. Straighten your arms to raise yourself back up into your starting position. Keep your elbows in tight – they shouldn't be bowing outwards. Repeat this exercise for 1 minute.

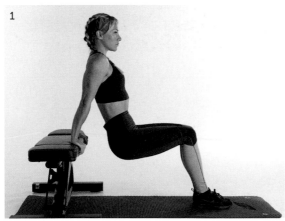
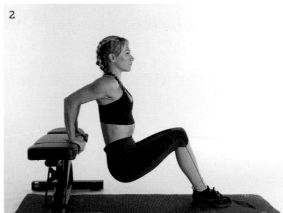

> **REST: 1 MINUTE**
> **REPEAT EXERCISES 1–4 AND REST x 5 TIMES**
> **TOTAL: 25 MINUTES**

HIIT MONDAY + WEDNESDAY + FRIDAY

HIIT CARDIO
BURPEES: ½ MINUTE » REST: 1½ MINUTES
REPEAT x 13 TIMES » 100% EFFORT!
TOTAL: 26 MINUTES

HIIT » BURPEES
100% EFFORT!

Stand up straight with your feet together and your arms down by your sides. »» Come down into a crouch and place your palms flat on the ground in front of you »» Put your body weight on your hands and jump your legs backwards, so you are in a plank position but resting on your hands, not on your elbows. »» Jump your legs back in, knees to your chest, to return to your crouch position. »» Finally, explode up into the air in a jump, landing back in your starting position. »» Continue this movement for ½ minute at 100% effort, then rest for 1½ minutes. Repeat 13 times.

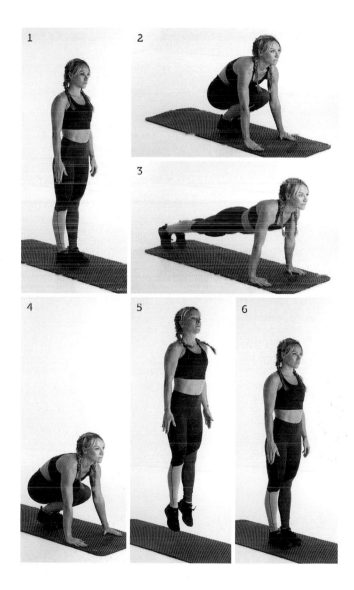

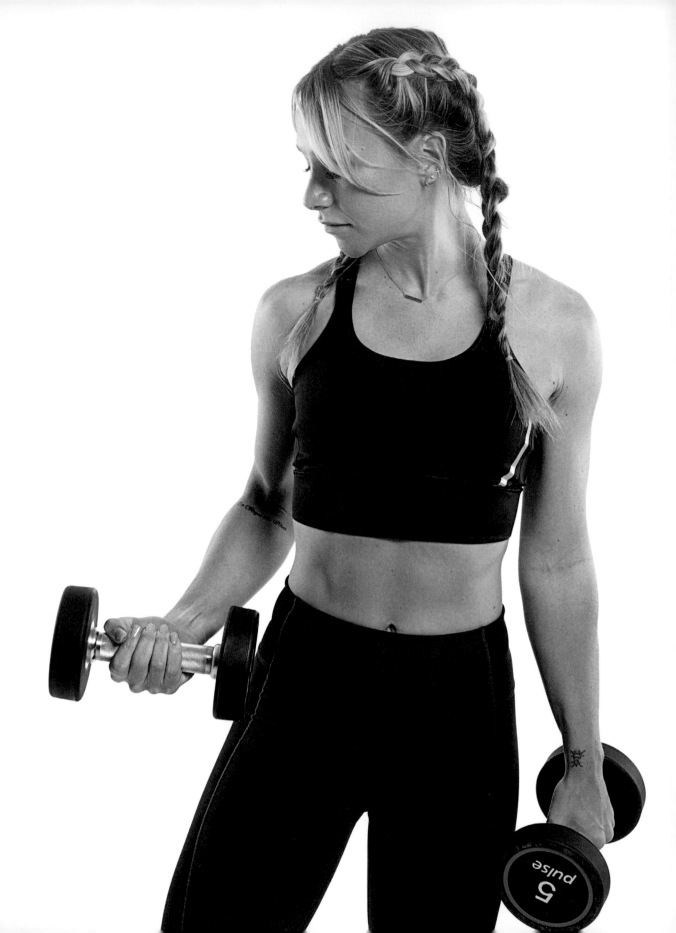

THE
GYM
PLAN

THE GYM DIET PLAN

In the GYM PLAN you have a weekly *and* a daily carb cycle, structured as follows:

>> 5 days low calorie via low-carb intake. (However, there will always be post-weightlifting carb meals for fuel, results and recovery.)

>> 2 days higher calorie via high-carb intake (re-feed).

Your WEEKLY food intake will look like this:

Monday – Low-carb Meals and Snacks (1 low-carb meal to be replaced with 1 high-carb meal post weightlifting)

Tuesday – Low-carb Meals and Snacks (1 low-carb meal to be replaced with 1 high-carb meal post weightlifting)

Wednesday – Low-carb Meals and Snacks (1 low-carb meal to be replaced with 1 high-carb meal post weightlifting)

Thursday – Low-carb Meals and Snacks (1 low-carb meal to be replaced with 1 high-carb meal post weightlifting)

Friday – Low-carb Meals and Snacks

Saturday – High-carb Meals and Snacks only (+1 carbohydrate snack)

Sunday – High-carb Meals and Snacks only (+1 carbohydrate snack)

Your MONDAY – FRIDAY intake will look like this:

1. Breakfast
2. Snack
3. Lunch
4. Snack
5. Dinner

Your SATURDAY + SUNDAY intake will look like this:

1. Breakfast
2. Snack
3. Lunch
4. Snack
5. Dinner
+
1 carbohydrate snack

>> You can eat these in any order you prefer, but you must eat *every single* meal and snack *daily*.

>> I also want you to make sure you **always eat a carbohydrate- and protein-based meal as soon as possible after any weightlifting session.**

Use the tables on pages 23–31 to build your own meals, or go to pages 152–213 for my recipes.

Monday – Friday

1. BREAKFAST
CHOOSE
1 protein option
1 fat option
1 veg option
OR
1 low-carb breakfast recipe

2. SNACK*
1 protein option
*Men to replace with 1 **low** carb meal

3. LUNCH
CHOOSE
1 protein option
1 fat option
1 veg option
OR
1 low-carb lunch or dinner recipe

4. SNACK*
1 protein option
*Men to replace with 1 **low**-carb meal

5. DINNER
CHOOSE
1 protein option
1 fat option
1 veg option
OR
1 low-carb lunch or dinner recipe

♂ Men must replace both daily snack options with **low-carb** meal options to ensure they hit an appropriate caloric count.

POST WEIGHTLIFTING
*Replace 1 **low**-carb meal with 1 **high**-carb meal*
CHOOSE
1 protein option
1 carb option
1 veg option
OR
1 high-carb recipe

Saturday + Sunday

1. BREAKFAST
CHOOSE
1 protein option
1 carb option
1 veg option
OR
1 high-carb breakfast recipe

2. SNACK*
1 protein option
*Men to replace with 1 **high**-carb meal

3. LUNCH
CHOOSE
1 protein option
1 carb option
1 veg option
OR
1 high-carb lunch or dinner recipe

4. SNACK*
1 protein option
*Men to replace with 1 **high**-carb meal

5. DINNER
CHOOSE
1 protein option
1 carb option
1 veg option
OR
1 high-carb lunch or dinner recipe

6. SNACK*
1 carbohydrate snack
*Men to replace with 1 **high**-carb meal

♂ Men must replace all three daily snack options with **high-carb** meal options to ensure they hit an appropriate calorie count.

TELL ME WHY...

» Five days in a calorie deficit (via carb depletion) will inevitably lead to a loss.

» Implementing two consecutive weekly re-feeds (via carb increases):

> Will feed your muscle, allowing you to refuel, recover and continue to train hard over the course of the next few days.

> The first re-feed will *halt* the drastic drop in hormonal and metabolic functions that are inevitable when implementing a low-calorie, fat-loss phase. This drop in hormonal and metabolic function is what leads to the infamous plateau.

> The second re-feed will ramp your hormonal and metabolic levels back up, allowing you to re-enter your depletion and continue to lose effectively, week on week, until you are ready to end *The Fat-Loss Blitz*.

Why am I implementing post-weightlifting carbs?

» While *growing* muscle is unlikely in a calorie deficit, you should at least be trying to hold on to the muscle you have. By eating a meal of protein and carbs as soon as possible post-lift, you are feeding your muscle, fuelling your muscle and encouraging your muscle to hang around.

» Recovery is key. You are encouraging your muscle to rebuild and recover, and you are helping yourself to go into that next session a little bit better off.

Additional benefits of the 5/2 SPLIT:

» A lot of my Blitzers take part in group sports, and teams tend to play at the weekends. These weekend re-feeds are a great way to go out there fully fuelled for a game and recover in the hours afterwards.

» Most of us have social events at the weekends. While you are not permitted to 'cheat' or drink alcohol on *The Fat-Loss Blitz*, having two higher calorie and carb days can make going out for meals seem a little less intimidating.

THE GYM TRAINING PLAN

The first thing I need to flag is that while this may be the Gym Plan, I have deliberately kept it simple so that Blitzers who want to progress to this point can transition as easily as possible.

The illustrations should help you recognise which machines and weights you need for each exercise and how to use them.

If you are ever unsure, though, the gym instructors and personal trainers on the gym floor are employed to show members how to use the equipment, so never be too shy to ask. They will be happy to show you.

Alternatively, YouTube is a great resource for training demonstrations and finding out how best to use a machine or weight. You will find a multitude of options as soon as you type in 'squat technique', for example.

For those of you who are slightly more experienced in the gym, while this plan may avoid 'bro sets' (super, tri, giant and pyramid sets), it is still designed to hit *every* area of your body effectively (legs, glutes, back, abs, shoulders, chest and arms), using different weights (free weights/machines etc.) and various training techniques (isometric holds, compound movements etc.) in order to get you *the best* aesthetic results possible.

You will be training different parts of the body on different days of the week. Training days also change during the course of the 4 weeks. This way, you will be training your body evenly *and* ensuring great aesthetic results en route.

The sets and reps range is 4 sets of 12 reps. This means you perform the movement 12 times, rest for 1 minute, then repeat the 12 reps and rest 3 more times. I have chosen this range because I want you to work your muscle and optimise your energy output, getting you the best possible results in terms of fat loss and body transformation.

While I do want you to follow my plan as closely as possible, I also know from experience that *most* people who have a long-standing love affair with weightlifting already know what works well for them. For example, while I keep squats in my lower body days because they are a great compound exercise, I certainly have never *felt* them work my glutes or *seen* them do so, either.

I have had countless people tell me that I should perform my lateral raises more horizontally, but when I do this, it takes the burn *out* of my deltoid and *into* my trapezius.

What I'm trying to say is that we all know when and where we feel something, and we all know what does and doesn't work for us personally. So, while it *can be* extremely helpful to receive and/or implement a new training plan, do feel free to cherry pick and/or edit the sessions.

BUT make sure that you:
>> Train your body evenly throughout the week (don't just focus on legs, for example).
>> Stick to the minimum cardio times *and* minimum training days.

Any day without training is a day of rest.

Newbies, please be aware that only you know what weight you can lift. It is 100% subjective and dependent on your own strength. A weight that challenges me would do absolutely nothing for my partner. A weight that challenges a beginner would probably not do much for me.

Everybody is different.

I want you to choose a weight that allows you to complete every set and rep, while making sure that by the last few reps you are really struggling.

Weightlifting is very subjective.
Only you can say what weight you should lift or where you feel the contraction. The right weight for you is one that really challenges you by the last few reps. And, as long as you are conscious of form and you lift safely, if you need to alter your position slightly, then do so. Personally, I have to perform almost every lower body exercise with a wide stance, otherwise my quads take over and exhaust halfway through the session. Finally, don't try to run before you can walk. Focus on form and perfecting the exercise *before* you try to increase the weight.

TELL ME WHY...

The first thing you'll notice is that you are doing:

4 SETS of 12 REPS

Normally when I'm gaining muscle, I try to go as heavy as I can while completing 3 sets of 8 reps.

A lot of the time I'll do pyramid sets that gradually increase in weight, so I can start on that final higher weight the following week and hit PBs for as long as possible.

However, when I am trying to shed fat, this structure changes somewhat.

Why?

It is nearly impossible to gain muscle when you are in a fat-loss phase. Your calories are too low, your cardio is too high and, most importantly, *gaining muscle is no longer the goal*.

That being said, 'use it or lose it' is a rule I train by, so I continue to use my muscle, just in a slightly more appropriate format for a fat-loss goal.

Doing 4 sets of 12 – while still going as heavy as you can – is going to have a much better effect on your fat- and calorie-burning priorities, while encouraging your body to continue to use and keep its muscle mass.

The second thing you'll notice is that you are doing HIIT twice a week, *only* on lower body days.

HIIT is great but there is a time and place for this form of cardio. It causes serious stress on the body and, when overdone, it can actually hinder your recovery, progress and results.

The ideal time to implement HIIT is when your body is already under unavoidable training stress... in other words, leg day.

You will be working your body **hard** on lower body days, so that's the perfect time to utilise high intensity interval training.

Another thing you'll notice is that I encourage you to take Fridays off. Friday is your last calorie deficit day before your first re-feed of the week on Saturday. Come Thursday/Friday, you're likely to feel a little sore and/or tired, so a rest day as close as possible to your first re-feed is really going to help.

Six days training a week is a lot, so if you need to take an extra rest day then do. However, try to keep it as close as possible to that first re-feed day when your body will need it most and recover best.

Finally, you'll see that as the weeks progress, so does your cardio. This weekly cardio increase is to ensure that you continue to progress throughout.

Monday + Thursday

WARM UP (SEE PAGES 42–51)

LOWER BODY

EXERCISES 1–6: x 4 SETS x 12 REPS

followed by

HIIT CARDIO (SEE PAGE 106)

ANY CARDIO MACHINE OR BURPEES: ½ MINUTE »
REST: 1½ MINUTES
REPEAT x 10 TIMES » **20 MINUTES**
100% EFFORT!

COOL DOWN (SEE PAGES 42–51)

If you are new to lifting, start with a light weight. If you are used to lifting, start with a weight that you know you can manage, but that will challenge you.

The Smith machine is not only great for beginners, it is also a great way for more experienced lifters to play around with their squat technique, from feet together, to hip width, to wide stance. The more you can vary the machines you use and the ranges you try, the better you will understand and train your body effectively.

LOWER BODY MONDAY + THURSDAY

1 SQUATS ON SMITH MACHINE x 4 sets x 12 reps

Make sure the weight is the same on each side of the bar. »» Find the centre of the horizontal bar and duck underneath it, so the bar is resting across your shoulders. »» Place your feet hip-width apart, or slightly further if that is a more comfortable squat position for you, and make sure your toes are either pointing forwards or slightly outwards, whichever is more comfortable. »» Take hold of the bar either side of your shoulders and unhook the bar from the machine – keep it unhooked using your grip. »» Standing up straight and bending only at the hips and knees, come down into a low squat before pushing back up through your heels to a standing position, squeezing your glutes as you do so. »» Take a breath and repeat this movement for the full amount of sets and reps.

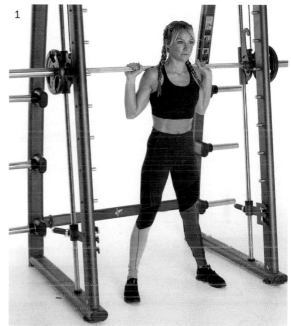

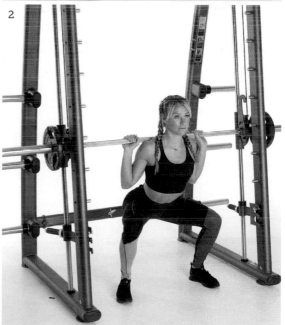

2 SPLIT SQUATS ON SMITH MACHINE x 4 sets x 12 reps

If you are new to lifting, you may not need to add a weight as the exercise is challenging unweighted. If you do add weight, make sure it is the same on each side of the bar. »» Place a bench about 0.5m behind you, so you are sandwiched between the Smith and the bench. »» Find the centre of the horizontal bar and duck underneath it, so the bar is resting across your shoulders. »» Place one foot up on the bench behind you, resting top down. Make sure the toes of your standing foot are pointing forwards. »» Place your hands either side of your shoulders and unhook the bar from the machine – keep it unhooked using your grip. »» Standing up straight and bending only at the hip and knee, come down into a low squat before pushing back up through your heel to a standing position. »» Take a breath and repeat on the other leg. Continue for the full amount of sets and reps.

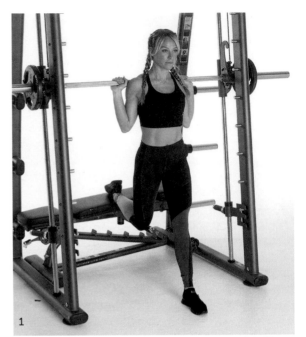

1

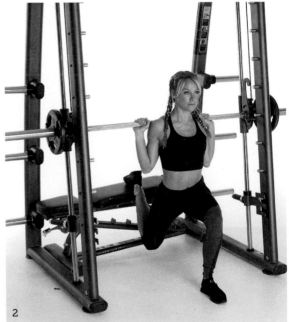

2

3 DEADLIFTS WITH OLYMPIC BAR x 4 sets x 12 reps

Find the Deadlift platform (this will look like a slightly raised mat or wooden area). Place the Olympic bar horizontally in front of your feet. Stand up straight with your feet hip-width apart, toes pointing forwards. »» Keeping your back straight and bending only at the hips and knees, crouch down so your hands are able to reach the bar. Grasp the bar either side of your legs, placing one hand overhand grip and the other underhand grip (whichever is more comfortable is fine). »» Once you have a good grip, stand up straight, pushing down through your heels as you do so. As you come into a fully vertical standing position, squeeze your buttocks at the top of the movement. »» Keeping the bar against your legs, slowly allow it to pull you back down to the ground again, keeping your back straight and bending only at the hips and knees at all times »» Allow the bar to hit the floor, take a breath and repeat the lift for the full amount of sets and reps.

1

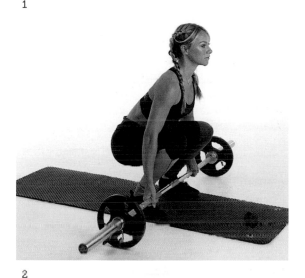

2

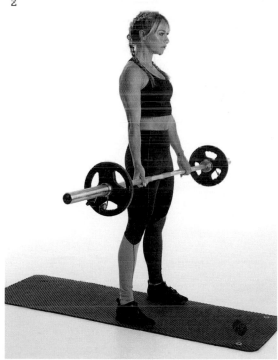

4 HIP THRUSTS ON SMITH MACHINE
x 4 sets x 12 reps

If you are new to lifting, you may not need to add a weight as this exercise is challenging unweighted. If you would like to try a weight, make sure it is the same on each side of the bar. »» Place a bench about 0.5m behind you, so you are sandwiched between the Smith and the bench. »» Lower the bar so it is about 30cm off the ground. »» Sit down between the bar and the bench, facing the bar and resting your upper back and shoulder blades on the edge of the bench. Place a bar pad (a black, cushioned tube) around the centre of the horizontal bar. Place your feet hip-width apart and keep your toes pointing forwards or slightly outwards. Place your hips underneath the cushion and your hands either side of your hips. »» Unhook the bar from the machine – keep it unhooked using your grip – and thrust up into the air, through your glutes, squeezing them tight at the top of the movement. Hold this position for a few seconds before coming back down until your buttocks are just above the ground. »» Take a breath and repeat the movement for the full amount of sets and reps.

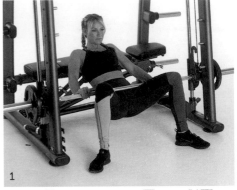

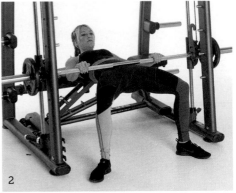

5 LEG PRESS ON MACHINE
x 4 sets x 12 reps

Sit down on the machine and place your feet hip-width apart on the plate in front of you (or slightly further apart if that is more comfortable). Keep your toes pointing upwards, or slightly outwards, whichever you prefer. »» Pushing through the flats of your feet, slowly and gently push the plate away from your lower body. »» Using the handles either side of the chair, move the ledge that is holding the plate in place. Once the plate is free, slowly let it come towards you until you cannot retreat your legs any further. »» At this point, slowly push the plate away until you are back in your starting position. Never lock your knees out, you should always keep a slight bend in them when performing any lower body lift. »» Take a breath and repeat this movement for the full amount of sets and reps.

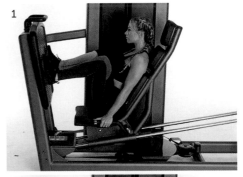

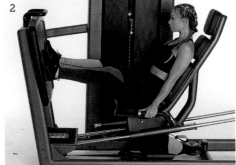

6 DONKEY KICK BACKS ON SMITH MACHINE
x 4 sets x 12 reps

Place a thick mat directly underneath the Smith bar. Make sure the weight is the same on each side of the bar. »» Kneel on the mat slightly in front of the bar and get down on all fours. »» Place the ball of your right foot under the bar and push up a little, then roll the bar back a little using the ball of your foot, and it will unhook itself. This needs a little skill and it may take a few sessions until you can do it seamlessly, but you will get there. »» Slowly and gently bring your knee down towards the mat and then push up until your leg is almost fully extended, always keeping a slight bend in the knee. »» Take a breath and repeat this movement for the full amount of sets and reps on each leg.

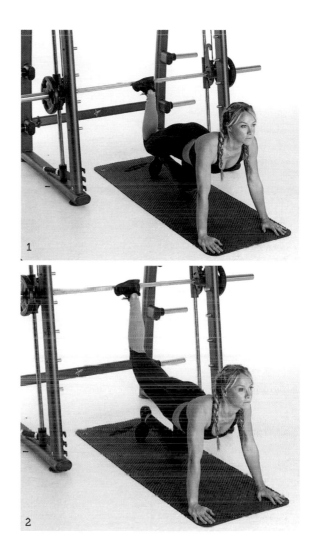

Donkey Kick Backs on the Smith machine are tricky at first, but after a few attempts you will unhook the bar with ease. Don't forget, there is always an alternative way to do every exercise – ankle weights or DKBs on the cable machine (performed standing) are both great alternatives.

HIIT CARDIO
ANY CARDIO MACHINE OR BURPEES: ½ MINUTE » REST: 1½ MINUTES
REPEAT x 10 TIMES » **100% EFFORT!**
TOTAL: 20 MINUTES

HIIT » BURPEES
100% EFFORT!

Stand up straight with your feet together and your arms down by your sides. »» Come down into a crouch and place your palms flat on the ground in front of you. »» Put your body weight on your hands and jump your legs backwards, so you are in a plank position but resting on your hands, not on your elbows. »» Jump your legs back in, knees to your chest, to return to your crouch position. »» Finally, explode up into the air in a jump, landing back in your starting position. »» Continue this movement for ½ minute at 100% effort, then rest for 1½ minutes. Repeat 10 times.

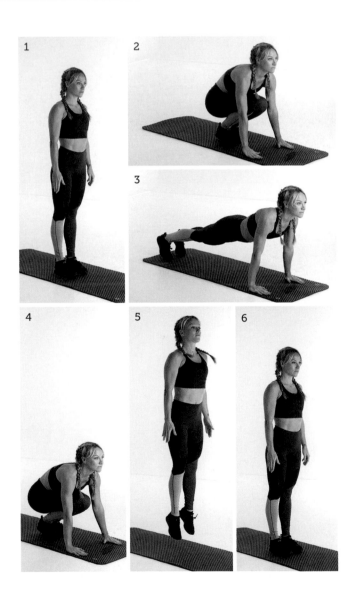

Tuesday + Saturday
WARM UP (SEE PAGES 42–51)
UPPER BODY
EXERCISES 1–6: x 4 SETS x 12 REPS
followed by
LOW–MODERATE INTENSITY CARDIO
ANY CARDIO MACHINE OR SWIMMING
FOR **20 MINUTES**
COOL DOWN (SEE PAGES 42–51)

1 CHEST PRESS ON BENCH x 4 sets x 12 reps

You will need a bench as well as dumbbells for this exercise. Make sure the dumbbell weight is the same in each hand. »» Sit on the bench with your feet flat on the floor on either side and grip the dumbbells in your hands, resting them on your thighs. »» Lie down on the bench and pull the dumbbells up so they are just above either side of your chest, making sure they are now horizontal. »» Slowly push the dumbbells up until your arms are fully extended, bringing them together at the peak of the lift so they lightly touch. »» Slowly bring the dumbbells back down to the starting position. Take a breath and repeat this movement for the full amount of sets and reps.

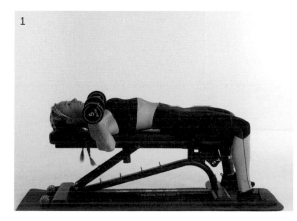
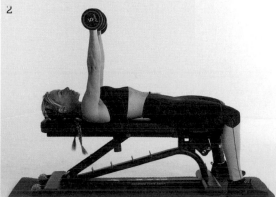

2 CHEST FLY WITH DUMBBELLS ON BENCH x 4 sets x 12 reps

You will need a bench as well as dumbbells for this exercise. Make sure the weight is the same in each hand. »» Sit on the bench with your feet flat on the floor on either side and grip the dumbbells in your hands, resting them on top of your thighs. »» Lie down on the bench. Keeping the dumbbells vertical in your grip, extend your arms out either side of your body at chest height. »» Then, as if you are hugging a beach ball, and keeping a slight bend in your elbows, bring the dumbbells together above your body. »» Slowly bring the dumbbells back down to the starting position. Take a breath and repeat this move for the full amount of sets and reps.

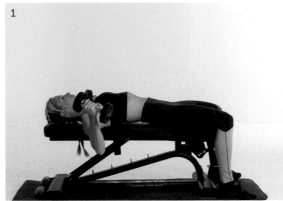

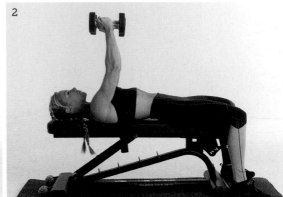

3 SHOULDER PRESS WITH DUMBBELLS x 4 sets x 12 reps

Grab two dumbbells and stand up straight with your feet hip-width apart and your toes pointing forwards. Grip the dumbbells using an overhand grip and allow them to hang in front of your hips. »» Swiftly swing them up so they are braced in front of your shoulders and, when you are ready, push them up above your head. As your arms come up to full extension, allow them to touch together gently in the air. »» Hold them there for a second, then slowly bring them back down to shoulder height. »» Take a deep breath and repeat this movement for the full amount of sets and reps.

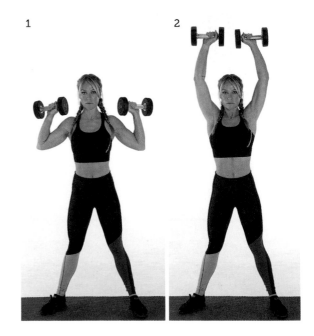

4 LATERAL RAISES WITH DUMBBELLS x 4 sets x 12 reps

Let me first start by saying that lateral raises are hard as your lateral muscles are very small, so if you are new to lifting, it will be a long time before you can increase the weight above what I call 'baby weight'. Make sure the weight is the same in each hand. »» Stand up straight with your knees slightly bent, your feet together and your toes pointing forwards. Grip the dumbbells in front of your crotch, lightly touching each other. Lean ever so slightly forward with your upper body, keeping an ever-so-slight arch in your lower back. »» Keeping a slight bend in your elbows and bowing them outwards slightly, slowly and gradually raise the dumbbells out either side of you, until your arms are horizontal, like an eagle in flight. »» Hold this position for a fraction of a second, then slowly bring your arms back down to your starting position. »» Take a breath and repeat this movement for the full amount of sets and reps.

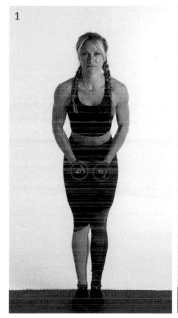
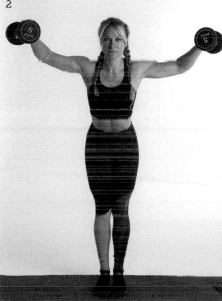
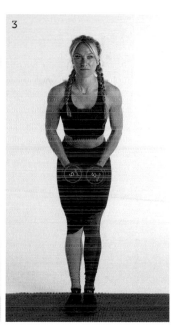

UPPER BODY TUESDAY + SATURDAY

5 FRONT RAISES WITH DUMBBELLS x 4 sets x 12 reps on each arm

As with lateral raises, the muscles worked by front raises are very small, so if you are new to lifting, it will be a long time before you can increase the weight above what I call 'baby weight'. Make sure the weight is the same in each hand. »» Stand up straight with your feet hip-width apart and your toes pointing forwards. Grip the dumbbells horizontally, using an overhand grip, and allow them to hang together in front of your crotch. »» Keeping your back straight at all times, take a deep breath and slowly raise one of the dumbbells. Keep a slight bend in your elbow as you do so. Hold the dumbbell in its raised position for a fraction of a second, then slowly bring it back down. »» Repeat with the alternate arm. »» Continue this movement alternately for the full amount of sets and reps.

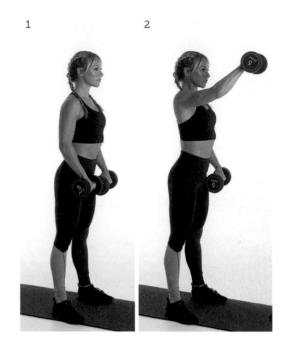

1 2

6 BENT OVER ROWS WITH DUMBBELLS x 4 sets x 12 reps on each arm

Place a dumbbell on the floor on the left-hand side of a bench. »» Keeping your left foot on the ground and your toes pointing forwards, place your right knee in the centre of the bench, then bend over and grip the top of the bench with your right hand. »» Keeping your back straight, slowly pick up the dumbbell with your left hand, making sure to keep your arm in tight to your body as you do so. »» Pull the dumbbell up into your armpit region and hold the dumbbell there for a fraction of a second, then slowly bring it back down to extend your arm. »» Continue this movement for the full amount of sets and reps, then repeat with alternate arm.

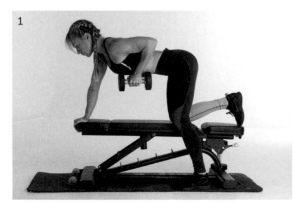

1

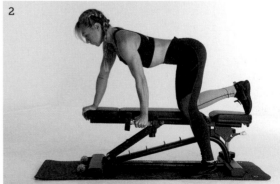

2

Wednesday + Sunday

WARM UP (SEE PAGES 42–51)
ABS
EXERCISES 1–6: x 1 SET TO EXHAUST
followed by
LOW–MODERATE INTENSITY CARDIO
ANY CARDIO MACHINE OR SWIMMING
FOR 20 MINUTES
COOL DOWN (SEE PAGES 42–51)

1 PLANK x 1 hold to exhaust

You may need a mat or cushion for your elbows during this exercise. Lie on your front with your feet hip-width apart, resting your toes against the top of the mat. Rest on your elbows and keep your forearms flat against the mat. Make sure your elbows are below your shoulders. Pushing against your toes and forearms, raise your body up into an elevated plank. *Do not* allow your spine to curve, either concavely or convexly – you want a straight back. Hold this position to exhaust. If you are struggling, feel free to transfer your weight from one foot to another, essentially shuffling your feet while holding the plank position.

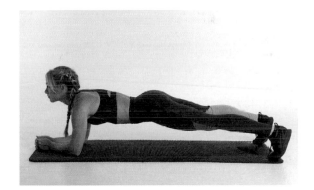

2 SIDE PLANK
x 1 set to exhaust

You may need a mat or cushion for this exercise. Lie on your side and prop your upper body up on your forearm (with a cushion underneath, if desired). Raise your outside hip up into the air and simultaneously push against your forearm and feet. Once one side of your body is in a rigid, straight line, engage your core and hold this position to exhaust. Repeat on the other side.

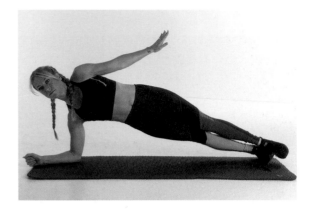

3 HEEL TAPS
x 1 set to exhaust

You may need a mat or a soft surface to cushion your back for this exercise. Lie on your back with your knees bent and your feet on the floor hip-width apart. Doing a very slight abdominal crunch so your upper back is slightly raised off the ground, stretch out your hands and move slowly to your right and left, repetitively, touching the outsides of your feet as you do so. Continue to perform this exercise to exhaust.

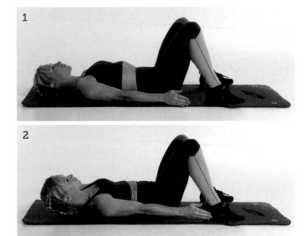

4 BICYCLES
x 1 set to exhaust

You may need a mat or a soft surface for this exercise. Lie on your back with your knees bent and your feet flat on the floor. Keeping your knees and feet together, raise your lower body up off the ground so your legs are bent at a 90-degree angle. Place your hands up by the sides of your head, elbows bent and pointing towards your knees. Slowly come up into a slight abdominal crunch and move your right elbow to your left knee, followed by your left elbow to your right knee. Continue to perform this exercise fluidly to exhaust.

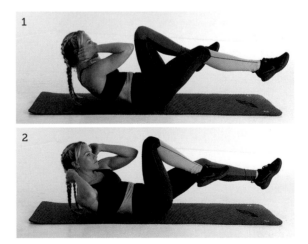

5 CRUNCHES ON MAT
x 1 set to exhaust

You will need a mat or a soft surface for this exercise. Lie on your back with your knees bent and your feet flat on the floor. Keeping your knees and feet together, use your abdominal muscles to slowly crunch upwards. Slowly come back down. Repeat this movement to exhaust.

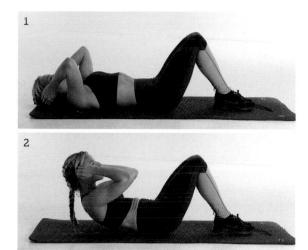

6 LEG RAISES ON MAT
x 1 set to exhaust

You will need a mat or a soft surface for this exercise. Lie on your back, extending your legs out fully and crossing your ankles. Keep your arms flat by your sides – feel free to hold on to the sides of the mat or on to a solid object behind your head to make this movement easier. Slowly raise your legs up into the air so they are vertical above your body, give a little upward thrust with your hips, raising your bottom off the floor, then slowly bring your legs back down to just above ground level. Repeat this movement to exhaust.

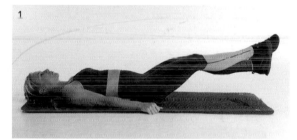

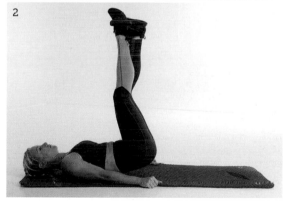

Monday + Thursday
WARM UP (SEE PAGES 42–51)
LOWER BODY
EXERCISES 1–6: x 4 SETS x 12 REPS
followed by
HIIT CARDIO (SEE PAGE 119)
ANY CARDIO MACHINE OR SQUAT JUMPS:
½ MINUTE » REST: 1½ MINUTES
REPEAT x 11 TIMES » **22 MINUTES**
100% EFFORT!
COOL DOWN (SEE PAGES 42–51)

If you are new to lifting, start with a light weight. If you are used to lifting, start with a weight that you know you can manage, but that will challenge you.

I know it may seem cruel to give you HIIT after your lower body workout, but your body will already be working hard to recover from those sessions, so you may as well throw in HIIT! For the rest of the week, you'll focus on more fat-burning cardio, with low-moderate intensity output.

1 WIDE STANCE SQUATS ON SMITH MACHINE
x 4 sets x 12 reps

Make sure the weight is the same on each side of the bar. »» Find the centre of the horizontal bar and duck underneath it, so the bar is now resting across your shoulders. »» Place your feet slightly wider than hip-width apart – as far as you are comfortable – and point your toes slightly outwards. »» Take hold of the bar either side of your shoulders and unhook it from the machine – keep it unhooked using your grip. »» Standing up straight, bending only at the hips and knees, come down into a low squat before pushing back up through your heels to a standing position, squeezing your glutes as you do so. »» Take a breath and repeat this movement for the full amount of sets and reps.

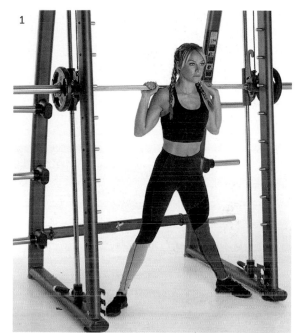

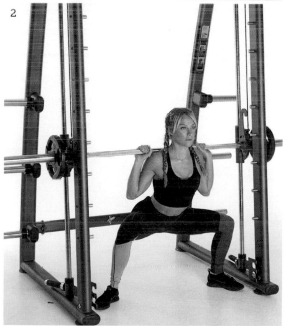

LOWER BODY MONDAY + THURSDAY

2 DONKEY SIDE KICKS x 4 sets x 12 reps on each leg

You may need a mat or a soft surface for this exercise. »» Get down on all fours. Make sure you keep your back straight – you don't want to do any damage by arching your spine during this exercise. »» Keeping the angular bend in your legs at all times, slowly raise one leg up and out to the side, until you feel the tension in your buttocks. »» Hold this position for 1 second before bringing your leg slowly back down to your starting position. »» Repeat with the opposite leg. »» Continue to perform the exercise alternately for 1 minute.

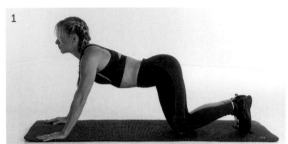
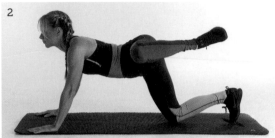

3 REVERSE LUNGES ON SMITH MACHINE x 4 sets x 12 reps on each leg

Make sure the weight is the same on each side of the bar. »» Find the centre of the horizontal bar and duck underneath it, so the bar is resting across your shoulders. Place your feet together with your toes pointing forwards. Place your hands on the bar either side of your shoulders and unhook the bar from the machine – keep it unhooked using your grip. »» Standing up straight, slowly step backwards with one of your feet, coming down into a low backwards lunge. »» As your knee is just about to touch the ground, push back up and return to your starting position. »» Repeat immediately with the alternate leg. »» Continue this movement alternately for the full amount of sets and reps.

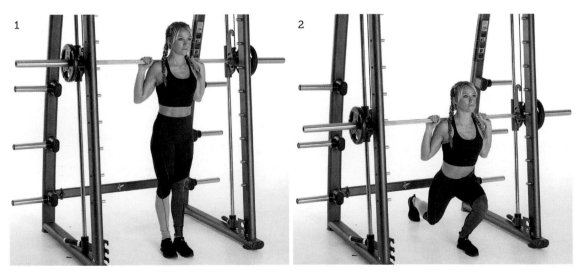

4 ROMANIAN DEADLIFTS WITH OLYMPIC BAR
x 4 sets x 12 reps

Place the Olympic bar in front of your feet. If you are new to lifting, you may not need to add a weight for this exercise as the Olympic bar is already weighted. If you would like to try a weight, make sure it is the same on each side of the bar. Also make sure you use bar clips whenever you use the Olympic bar, placed either side of the weight plate. »» Stand up straight with your feet hip-width apart and your toes pointing forwards. »» Keeping your back straight and bending only at the hips and knees, crouch down so your hands are now able to grasp the bar. Grasp it either side of your legs, placing one hand in an overhand grip, the other in an underhand grip (whichever hand is more comfortable is fine). »» Once you have a good grip on the bar, stand up straight, pushing down through your heels as you do so. As you come into a full standing position, squeeze your buttocks at the top of the movement. »» Pull your shoulders back, like there is a corset between your shoulder blades, and *keep them back* during this exercise. Engage your core and make sure to keep your entire core and back position solid throughout. »» Keeping the bar against your legs, slowly allow it to pull you down from the hips as far as your hamstrings will allow – sticking your bottom out as you go. »» Take a breath and return to your starting position. Repeat the lift for the full amount of sets and reps.

1

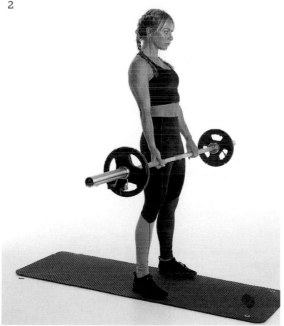

2

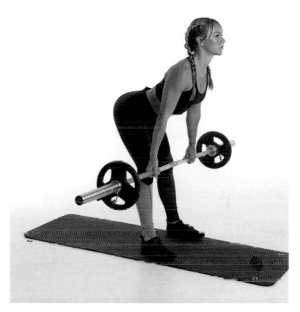

5 GLUTE BRIDGE HOLD ON SMITH MACHINE x 1 set to exhaust

If you are new to lifting, you may not need to add a weight as this exercise is challenging unweighted. If you would like to try a weight, make sure it is the same on each side of the bar. »» Lower the bar down so it is about 30cm off the ground and place a bar pad (a black, cushioned tube) around the centre of the horizontal bar. Lie down underneath the bar with your hips directly under the bar pad. »» With your knees pointing upwards at a 90-degree angle, place your feet hip-width apart, or slightly further if that is more comfortable, and keep your toes pointing forwards or slightly outwards, whichever you prefer. Place your hips underneath the cushion and your hands either side of your hips, gripping the bar. »» Unhook the bar from the machine – keep it unhooked using your grip – and thrust up into the air, through your glutes, squeezing them tight at the top of the movement. »» Hold to exhaust.

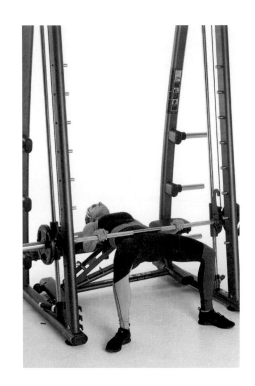

6 ABDUCTOR MACHINE x 4 sets x 12 reps

Sit on the machine and, using the prong at the side of the chair, alter the pads so that your knees are as close together as possible. »» Sit up straight and, using your knees, slowly push the pads outwards and squeeze your buttocks, engaging your glutes, as you do so (I like to do a little seated hip thrust to really engage my glutes here). »» Hold this position for a moment before slowly coming back into your starting position. »» Take a deep breath and repeat this movement for the full sets and reps.

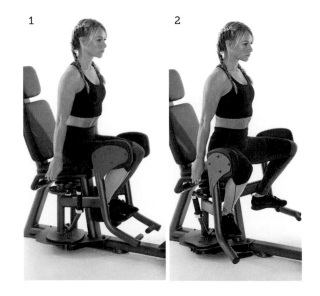

HIIT CARDIO
ANY CARDIO MACHINE OR SQUAT JUMPS: ½ MINUTE »
REST: 1½ MINUTES » REPEAT X 11 TIMES » 100% EFFORT!
TOTAL: 22 MINUTES

HIIT » SQUAT JUMPS 100% EFFORT!

Stand up straight with your feet hip-width apart. »» Extend your arms out in front of you and place one hand on top of the other – or place your hands on your hips, whichever is more comfortable. »» Keeping your back straight, lower yourself down into a deep squat by bending your knees. Instead of standing back up again from the squat, gently jump back into a standing position. The jump should be so gentle that you can maintain your form from the very start of the exercise to the next repetition. It should also be so gentle that you only come off the floor a little. Big dynamic jumps can damage your joints, so keep it gentle. »» Continue this movement for ½ minute at 100% effort then rest for 1½ minutes. Repeat 11 times.

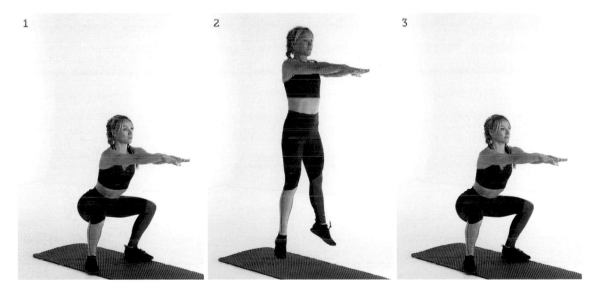

Tuesday + Saturday
WARM UP (SEE PAGES 42–51)
UPPER BODY
EXERCISES 1–6: x 4 SETS x 12 REPS
followed by
LOW–MODERATE INTENSITY CARDIO
ANY CARDIO MACHINE OR SWIMMING
FOR 25 MINUTES
COOL DOWN (SEE PAGES 42–51)

1 DUMBBELL PULLOVERS ON BENCH x 4 sets x 12 reps

››› Sit on the bench, legs either side of it, and grip the dumbbell (vertically) between your legs. ››› Lie down and, as you do so, raise the dumbbell up in the air, directly above your face. ››› Now adjust your grip by opening your hands, allowing the weight of the dumbbell to rest against the flats of your palms, gripping around its base with your fingers. ››› Allow the dumbbell to slowly and gently come behind you, so that it is both behind your head and behind the bench. ››› Slowly and gently, bring it back up into the air, above your face, into your starting position. ››› Take a deep breath and repeat this movement for the full amount of sets and reps.

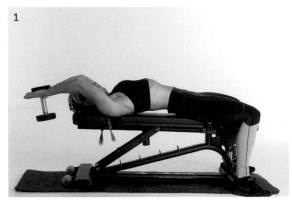
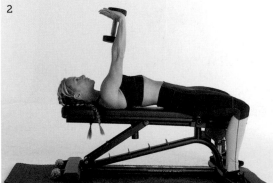

2 ASSISTED CLOSE GRIP PULL UPS ON MACHINE x 4 sets x 12 reps

Make sure the padded seat of the assisted machine is upright, ready for you to kneel on. »» Grip the bars above you that are closest together using an underhand grip. »» Place your knees on top of the padded seat. »» Slowly allow your body to drop down underneath the bars. »» Once your arms are fully extended, slowly pull yourself back up into a pull-up position. »» Hold this position for a second before allowing yourself to come back down again »» Take a deep breath and repeat this movement for the full amount of sets and reps.

1   2   3

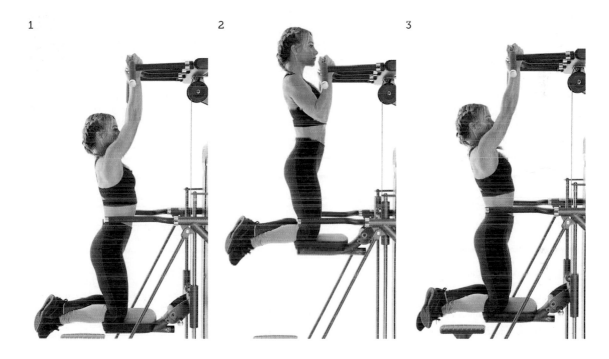

If you are new to lifting, place the toggle on one of the lowest, heaviest weight plates, to ensure you won't be pulling your entire body weight (this is what is meant by 'assisted'). If you are used to lifting, start with a weight that you know you can manage, but that will challenge you.

3 ASSISTED WIDE GRIP PULL UPS ON MACHINE
x 4 sets x 12 reps

Make sure the padded seat is upright. ››› Grip the bars that are furthest apart using an overhand grip and place your knees on top of the padded seat. ››› Slowly allow your body to drop down underneath the bars. Once your arms are fully extended, slowly pull yourself back up into a wide-grip pull-up position. ››› Hold this for a second before allowing yourself to come back down to your starting position. ››› Take a deep breath and repeat this movement for the full amount of sets and reps.

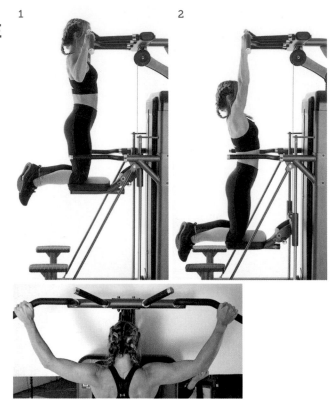

4 ASSISTED TRICEP DIPS ON MACHINE
x 4 sets x 12 reps

Make sure the padded seat is upright and the bars on either side of the machine are as close together as possible (they are often adjustable). ››› Grip the bars using an inverted grip and place your knees on top of the padded seat. ››› Keeping your elbows in tight to your sides, slowly allow your body to drop down. ››› When you have come down as far as possible, slowly push yourself back up, using your triceps. ››› Take a deep breath and repeat this movement for the full amount of sets and reps.

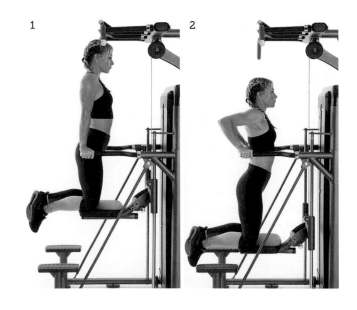

5 HYPEREXTENSIONS
x 4 sets x 12 reps

You will need a mat to cushion your front for this exercise. Lie face down on the mat and cross your ankles. »» Place your hands either side of your head and slowly bow your body back into a lower back crunch (another name for this exercise is a reverse sit up). »» Make sure you engage your glutes and core while doing this exercise. »» Hold this position for a few seconds then repeat the movement for the full amount of sets and reps.

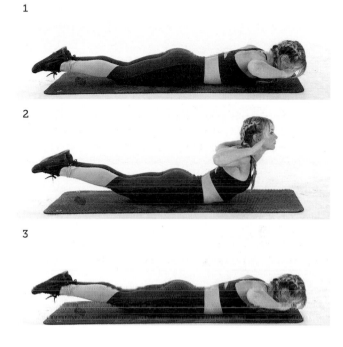

6 CLOSE GRIP ROWS ON MACHINE
x 4 sets x 12 reps

Sit down with your legs either side of the machine and grip the handles in front of you with an inverted grip. »» Take a deep breath and, slowly and gently, pull the handles into your chest. »» Hold the handles against yourself for a second, then slowly and gently let them pull you back out towards the starting position. »» Take a deep breath and repeat this movement for the full amount of sets and reps.

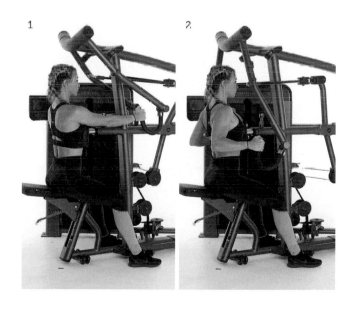

Wednesday + Sunday
WARM UP (SEE PAGES 42–51)
ABS
EXERCISES 1–6: x 1 SET TO EXHAUST
followed by
LOW–MODERATE INTENSITY CARDIO
ANY CARDIO MACHINE OR SWIMMING
FOR 25 MINUTES
COOL DOWN (SEE PAGES 42–51)

1 MOUNTAIN CLIMBERS x 1 set to exhaust

Lie on your front, feet hip-width apart, toes facing towards the floor. Place your hands by the sides of your chest, palms to the floor. Push yourself up using your hands and feet. Bring one knee up to your chest and then return it to the starting position. As you do this, switch legs. Repeat to exhaust.

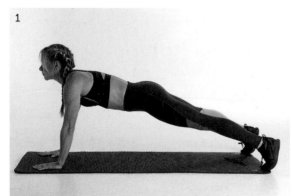
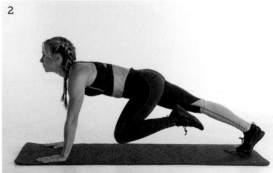

2 ELBOWS TO HAND PLANK
x 1 set to exhaust

You may need a mat or cushion for your
elbows during this exercise. Lie on your
front with your feet hip-width apart, resting
your toes against the top of the mat. Lean
on your elbows and keep your forearms flat
against the mat. Make sure your elbows are
below your shoulders. Pushing against your
toes and forearms, raise your upper body
into the air, one arm at a time, to rest on
your hands, so you form an elevated plank.
Do not allow your spine to curve, either
concavely or convexly. You want a straight
back. Come back down to rest on your
forearms, one arm at a time, and then push
back up on to your hands. Repeat to exhaust.

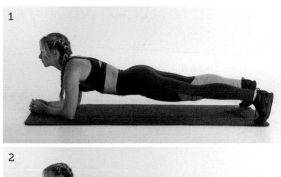

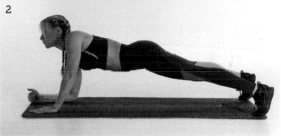

3 SIDE BENDS UNWEIGHTED
x 1 set to exhaust

Stand up straight with your feet hip-width
apart, your arms flat by your sides, and your
fingertips pointing down towards the floor.
Engage your core, tensing your mid-section
as if you are about to be punched in the
stomach. Slowly and in a controlled manner,
bend to one side as far as your natural range
will allow. Still tensing your stomach, use
your core to come back up to a straight,
standing position (again, do this slowly
and in a controlled manner). Repeat this
movement on the opposite side. Continue
to perform alternately to exhaust.

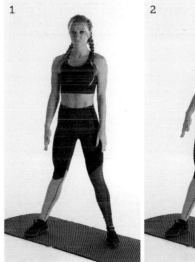

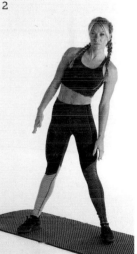

4 RUSSIAN TWISTS WITH WEIGHT PLATE x 1 set to exhaust

You will need a mat for this exercise. Sit upright on the mat, knees slightly bent and your ankles crossed in front of you. Raise your ankles up off the ground by 5cm or so and hold the weight out in front of your stomach. Slowly twist your abdominals and upper body to one side, allowing the weight to touch the mat beside your hips. Bring the weight back to the centre and repeat this move on the other side. Repeat this movement fluidly to exhaust.

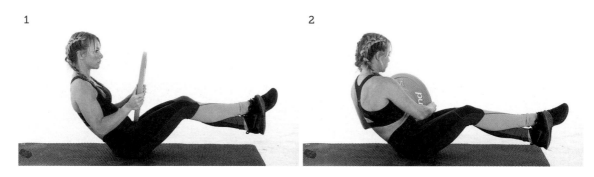

5 SIT UPS ON MAT x 1 set to exhaust

You will need a mat or a soft surface for this exercise. If you have never done ab exercises before, or you know you have a weak core, feel free to slide your feet under something to provide resistance – this will aid the sitting-up movement. Lie flat on your back and keep your knees bent, with your legs and feet together. Sit up, then gently lower yourself back down again. Repeat this movement to exhaust.

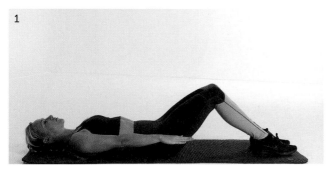
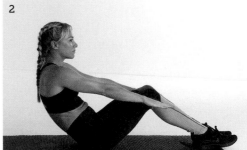

6 LEG RAISES ON MACHINE x 1 set to exhaust

Stand on the leg raise machine. Keep your back straight against the back pad and grip both the handles with an inverted grip. Let your legs dangle underneath you and cross your ankles. Slowly raise your legs up in front of you, then slowly allow them to come back down to your starting position. Repeat this move fluidly to exhaust.

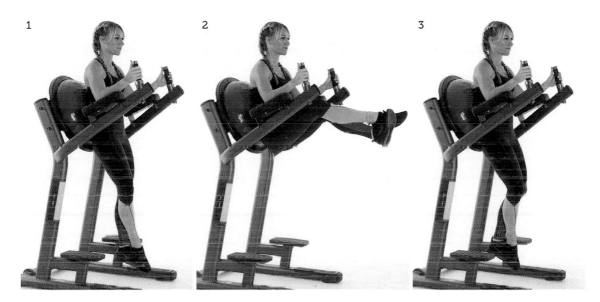

1   2   3

When I instruct x 1 set to exhaust,
I don't mean go until you can't be bothered
any more! I mean go until you exhaust and
your core cannot perform another rep.

Monday + Thursday

WARM UP (SEE PAGES 42–51)

LOWER BODY

EXERCISES 1–6: x 4 SETS x 12 REPS

followed by

HIIT CARDIO (SEE PAGE 133)

ANY CARDIO MACHINE OR MOUNTAIN CLIMBERS
½ MINUTE » REST: 1½ MINUTES
REPEAT x 12 TIMES » **24 MINUTES**
100% EFFORT!

COOL DOWN (SEE PAGES 42–51)

If you are new to lifting, start with a light weight. If you are used to lifting, start with a weight that you know you can manage, but that will challenge you.

Every week your HIIT will increase by 2 minutes. This is to ensure you continue to progress and see results. I also want you to make sure you always give your HIIT 100% effort, as this is how and why it works your metabolic rate so well.

1 BULGARIAN SPLIT SQUATS ON SMITH MACHINE
x 4 sets x 12 reps on each leg

You may not need to add a weight for this exercise as it is challenging unweighted. If you would like to try a weight, make sure it is the same on each side of the bar. »» Place the bench about 0.5m behind you, so you are sandwiched between the Smith and the bench. »» Find the centre of the horizontal bar and duck underneath it, so the bar is resting across your shoulders. »» Place one foot up on the bench behind you, resting top down. Make sure the toes of your standing foot are pointing forwards. »» Take hold of the bar either side of your shoulders and unhook the bar from the machine – keep it unhooked using your grip. »» Standing up straight and bending only at the hip and knee, come down into a low squat before pushing back up through your heel to a standing position. Take a breath and repeat on the other leg. Repeat for the full amount of sets and reps.

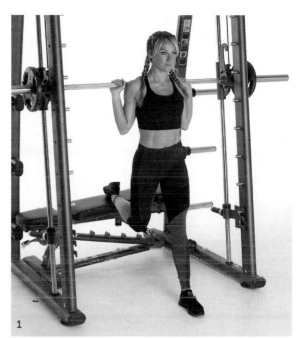

1

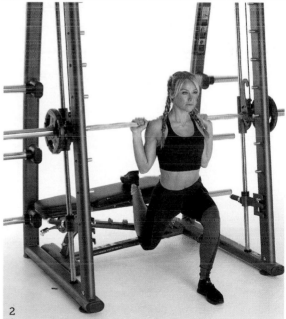

2

LOWER BODY MONDAY + THURSDAY

2 HIP THRUSTS ON SMITH MACHINE x 4 sets x 12 reps

If you are new to lifting, you may not need to add a weight as this exercise is challenging unweighted. If you would like to try a weight, make sure it is the same on each side of the bar. »» Place a bench about 0.5m behind you, so you are sandwiched between the Smith and the bench. »» Lower the bar so it is about 30cm off the ground. »» Sit down between the bar and the bench, facing the bar and resting your upper back and shoulder blades on the edge of the bench. Place a bar pad (a black, cushioned tube) around the centre of the horizontal bar. Place your feet hip-width apart and keep your toes pointing forwards or slightly outwards. Place your hips underneath the cushion and your hands either side of your hips. »» Unhook the bar from the machine – keep it unhooked using your grip – and thrust up into the air, through your glutes, squeezing them tight at the top of the movement. Hold this position for a few seconds before coming back down until your buttocks are just above the ground. »» Take a breath and repeat the movement for the full amount of sets and reps.

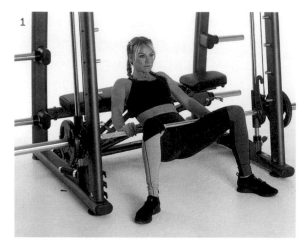

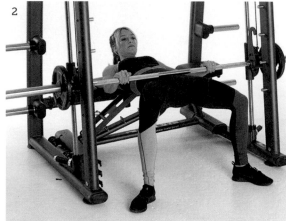

3 LEG CURLS ON MACHINE x 4 sets x 12 reps

Sit down on the leg curl machine, placing the backs of your ankles over the cushioned bar in front of you. »» You may need to adjust the chair so that your ankles sit comfortably on top of it. »» Slowly and gently push the cushioned bar down using your ankles and hamstrings. Then, slowly and gently, allow the bar to come back up to its starting position. »» Take a deep breath and repeat this movement for the full amount of sets and reps.

1   2

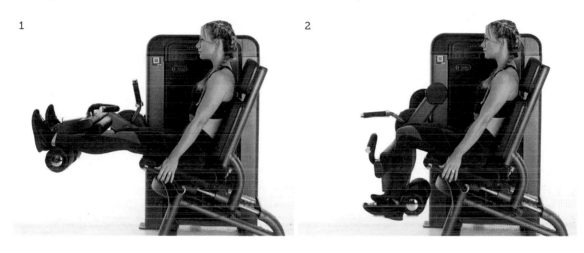

4 LEG EXTENSION ON MACHINE x 4 sets x 12 reps

Sit down on the leg extension machine, placing the fronts of your ankles under the cushioned bar in front of you. You may need to adjust the chair so that your ankles sit comfortably underneath it. »» Slowly and gently push the cushioned bar up using your ankles and quadriceps. Then, slowly and gently, allow the bar to come down to its starting position. »» Take a deep breath and repeat this movement for the full amount of sets and reps.

1   2

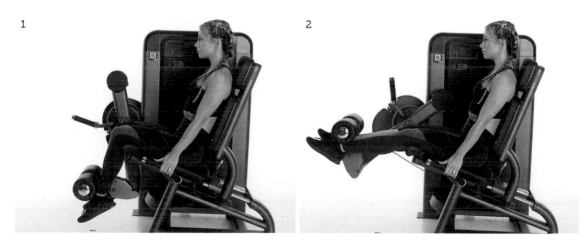

5 ABDUCTOR MACHINE
x 4 sets x 12 reps

Sit on the machine and, using the prong at the side of the chair, alter the pads so that your knees are as close together as possible. »» Sit up straight and, using your knees, slowly push the pads outwards and squeeze your buttocks, engaging your glutes, as you do so (I like to do a little seated hip thrust to really engage my glutes here). »» Hold this position for a moment before slowly coming back into your starting position. »» Take a deep breath and repeat this movement for the full sets and reps.

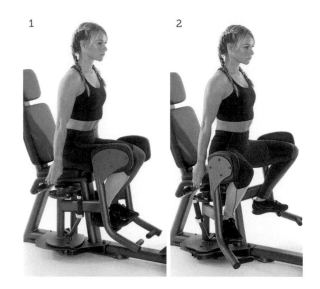

6 LEG PRESS ON MACHINE
x 4 sets x 12 reps

Make sure the weight is the same on each side of the bar. »» Sit down on the machine and place your feet hip-width apart on the plate in front of you (or slightly further apart if that is more comfortable). Keep your toes pointing upwards, or slightly outwards, whichever you prefer. »» Pushing through the flats of your feet, slowly and gently push the plate away from your lower body. »» Using the handles either side of the chair, move the ledge that is holding the plate in place. Once the plate is free, slowly let it come towards you until you cannot retreat your legs any further. »» At this point, slowly push the plate away until you are back in your starting position. Never lock your knees out, you should always keep a slight bend in them when performing any lower body lift. »» Take a breath and repeat this movement for the full amount of sets and reps.

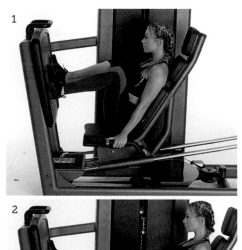

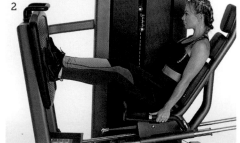

HIIT CARDIO
ANY CARDIO MACHINE OR MOUNTAIN CLIMBERS: 1/2 MINUTE »
REST: 1½ MINUTES » REPEAT X 12 TIMES » 100% EFFORT!
TOTAL: 24 MINUTES

HIIT »
MOUNTAIN CLIMBERS
100% EFFORT!

Lie on your front, feet hip-width apart, toes on the floor. » Place your hands by the sides of your chest, palms to the floor. » Push yourself up using your hands and feet. » Bring one knee up to your chest and then return it to the starting position. As you do this, switch legs. » Continue this movement for 1/2 minute at 100% effort then rest for 1½ minutes. Repeat 12 times.

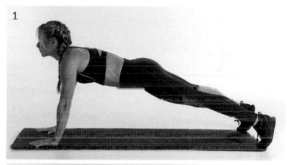

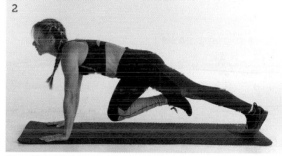

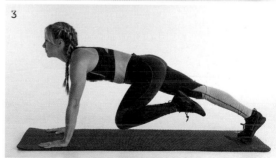

I don't care what cardio you choose for your HIIT, just make sure you give it 100%!

Tuesday + Saturday

WARM UP (SEE PAGES 42–51)

UPPER BODY

EXERCISES 1–6: x 4 SETS x 12 REPS

followed by

LOW–MODERATE INTENSITY CARDIO

ANY CARDIO MACHINE

FOR **25 MINUTES**

COOL DOWN (SEE PAGES 42–51)

You will find that you have to lift
'baby weights' when you train shoulders.
Don't be disheartened, it is simply because
the deltoid is a very small muscle,
so naturally it produces less force.

1 MILITARY PRESS WITH BARBELL
x 4 sets x 12 reps

Stand up straight with your feet hip-width apart and your toes pointing forwards. »» Grip the bar with your hands shoulder-width apart, using an overhand grip. »» Allow the bar to hang in front of your hips, then swiftly swing it up so that it is at chest height. »» Push the bar up above your head until your arms are fully extended. »» Hold the bar above your head for a second, then slowly bring it back down to chest height. »» Take a deep breath and repeat this movement for the full amount of sets and reps.

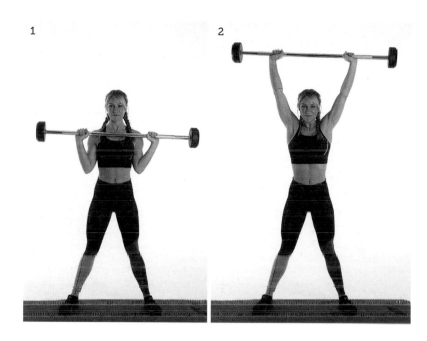

2 FRONT RAISES WITH WEIGHT PLATE
x 4 sets x 12 reps

Stand up straight with your feet hip-width apart. »» Grabbing the weight with both hands, hold it in front of your stomach. »» Extending your arms, bring the weight up in front of your chest, always keeping a slight bend in your elbows. »» Hold the weight for a second, then slowly bring it back down to stomach height. »» Take a deep breath and repeat this movement for the full amount of sets and reps.

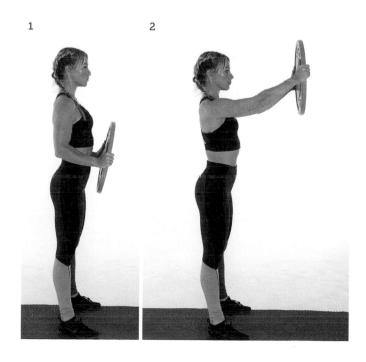

3 LATERAL RAISES WITH DUMBBELLS
x 4 sets x 12 reps

Make sure the weight is the same in each hand. »» Stand up straight with your knees slightly bent, your feet together and your toes pointed forwards. Grip the dumbbells in front of your crotch, lightly touching each other. Lean ever so slightly forward with your upper body, keeping an ever-so-slight arch in your lower back. »» Keeping a slight bend in your elbows and bowing them outwards slightly, slowly and gradually raise the dumbbells out either side of you, until your arms are horizontal, like an eagle in flight. »» Hold this position for a fraction of a second, then slowly bring your arms back down to your starting position. »» Take a breath and repeat this movement for the full amount of sets and reps.

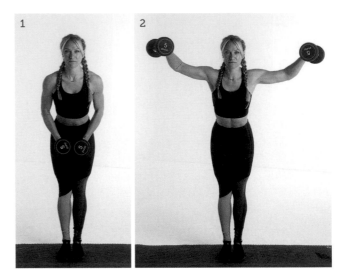

4 BENT OVER ROWS WITH BARBELL
x 4 sets x 12 reps

Stand up straight with your feet hip-width apart. Grabbing the weight with both hands, hold it in front of your stomach. »» Bring the weight up in front of your chest, always keeping a slight bend in your elbows. »» Hold the weight in front of you for a second, then slowly bring it back down to stomach height. »» Take a deep breath and repeat this movement for the full amount of sets and reps.

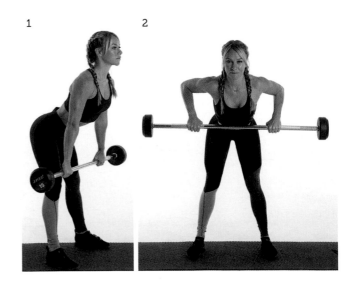

5 ASSISTED CLOSE GRIP PULL UPS ON MACHINE
x 4 sets x 12 reps

Make sure the padded seat is upright, ready for you to kneel on. »» Grip the bars above you that are closest together using an underhand grip. »» Place your knees on top of the padded seat, then slowly allow your body to drop down underneath the bars. »» Once your arms are fully extended, slowly pull yourself back up into a pull-up position. »» Hold this position for a second before allowing yourself to come back down again. »» Take a deep breath and repeat this movement for the full amount of sets and reps.

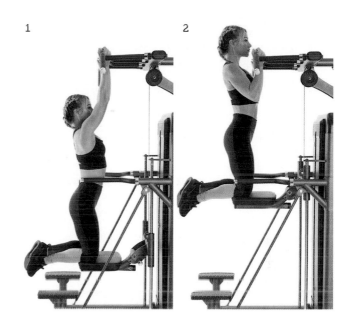

6 ASSISTED TRICEP DIPS ON MACHINE
x 4 sets x 12 reps

Make sure the padded seat is upright. »» Make sure the bars on either side of the machine are as close together as possible (they are often adjustable). »» Grip the bars using an inverted grip and place your knees on top of the padded seat. »» Keeping your elbows in tight to your sides, slowly allow your body to drop down. »» When you have come down as far as possible, slowly push yourself back up, using your triceps. »» Take a deep breath and repeat this movement for the full amount of sets and reps.

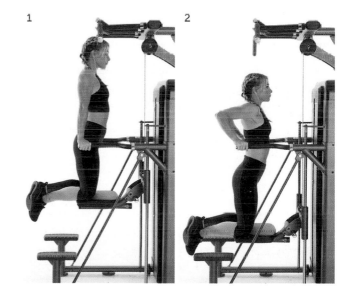

Wednesday + Sunday

WARM UP (SEE PAGES 42–51)

ABS

EXERCISES 1–6: x 1 SET TO EXHAUST

followed by

LOW–MODERATE INTENSITY CARDIO

ANY CARDIO MACHINE OR SWIMMING

FOR **25 MINUTES**

COOL DOWN (SEE PAGES 42–51)

1 PLANK x 1 hold to exhaust

You may need a mat or cushion for your elbows during this exercise. Lie on your front with your feet hip-width apart, resting your toes against the top of the mat. Rest on your elbows and keep your forearms flat against the mat. Make sure your elbows are below your shoulders. Pushing against your toes and forearms, raise your body up into an elevated plank. *Do not* allow your spine to curve, either concavely or convexly – you want a straight back. Hold this position to exhaust. If you are struggling, feel free to transfer your weight from one foot to another, essentially shuffling your feet while holding the plank position.

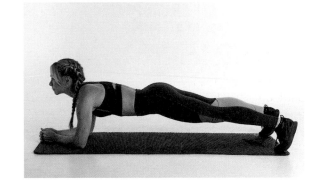

2 V SIT UPS WITH DUMBBELL ON MAT x 1 set to exhaust

You will need a mat for this exercise. Lie down, fully extended on the mat, gripping the weight in front of your chest, with your knees and ankles together in front of you. Extend your arms out above your head, so you are now fully stretched out, with the weight above your head. Using your arms and abdominals, slowly and gradually bring your upper body into a crunch, simultaneously lifting your legs up off the ground and into the air (your shins and the weight should meet half way). Slowly and gradually come back down into your starting position. Repeat this movement fluidly to exhaust.

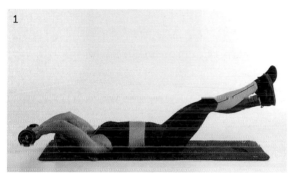
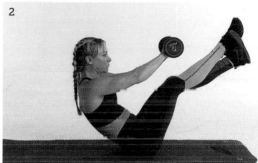

3 BICYCLES x 1 set to exhaust

You may need a mat or a soft surface for this exercise. Lie on your back with your knees bent and your feet flat on the floor. Keeping your knees and feet together, raise your lower body up off the ground so your legs are bent at a 90-degree angle. Place your hands up by the sides of your head, elbows bent and pointing towards your knees. Slowly come up into a slight abdominal crunch and move your right elbow to your left knee, followed by your left elbow to your right knee. Continue to perform this exercise fluidly to exhaust.

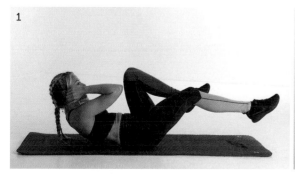
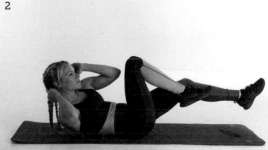

3 SIDE BENDS UNWEIGHTED x 1 set to exhaust

Stand up straight with your feet hip-width apart, your arms flat by your sides, and your fingertips pointing down towards the floor. Engage your core, tensing your mid-section as if you are about to be punched in the stomach. Slowly and in a controlled manner, bend to one side as far as your natural range will allow. Still tensing your stomach, use your core to come back up to a straight, standing position (again, do this slowly and in a controlled manner). Repeat this movement on the opposite side. Continue to perform alternately to exhaust.

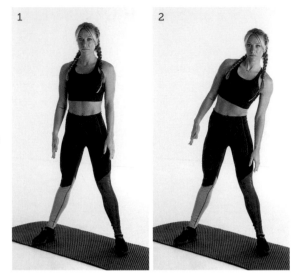

4 CRUNCHES ON MAT x 1 set to exhaust

You will need a mat or a soft surface for this exercise. Lie on your back with your knees bent and your feet flat on the floor. Keeping your knees and feet together, use your abdominal muscles to slowly crunch upwards. Slowly come back down. Repeat this movement to exhaust.

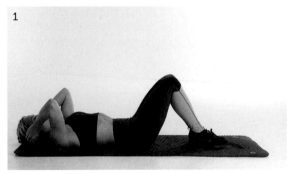
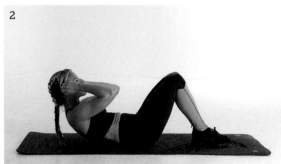

5 LEG RAISES ON MAT x 1 set to exhaust

You will need a mat or a soft surface for this exercise. Lie on your back, extending your legs out fully and crossing your ankles. Keep your arms flat by your sides – feel free to hold on to the sides of the mat or on to a solid object behind your head to make this movement easier. Slowly raise your legs up into the air so they are vertical above your body, give a little upward thrust with your hips, raising your bottom off the floor, then slowly bring your legs back down to just above ground level. Repeat this movement to exhaust.

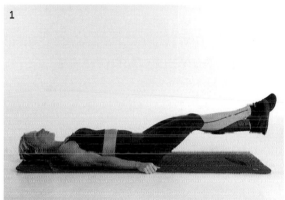
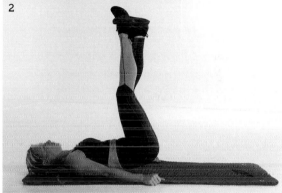

I have included ab work in the Gym Plan because training your core will assist your big, compound lifts (like squats) and vice versa. However, if you would like to swap some of your core sessions for weighted sessions, be my guest.

Monday + Thursday

WARM UP (SEE PAGES 42–51)

LOWER BODY

EXERCISES 1–6: x 4 SETS x 12 REPS

followed by

HIIT CARDIO (SEE PAGE 149)

ANY CARDIO MACHINE OR KETTLEBELL SWINGS

$\frac{1}{2}$ MINUTE » REST: $1\frac{1}{2}$ MINUTES

REPEAT x 13 TIMES » **26 MINUTES**

100% EFFORT!

COOL DOWN (SEE PAGES 42–51)

If you are new to lifting, start with a light weight. If you are used to lifting, start with a weight that you know you can manage, but that will challenge you.

Kettlebell swings (see page 149) are a great form of HIIT and resistance to boot. From your legs to your glutes, your core to your shoulders, there isn't much this movement won't do for your body transformation goals.

LOWER BODY

1 LEG EXTENSION ON MACHINE x 4 sets x 12 reps

Sit down on the leg extension machine, placing the fronts of your ankles under the cushioned bar in front of you. You may need to adjust the chair so that your ankles sit comfortably underneath it. »» Slowly and gently push the cushioned bar up using your ankles and quadriceps. Then, slowly and gently, allow the bar to come down to its starting position. »» Take a deep breath and repeat this movement for the full amount of sets and reps.

1
      2

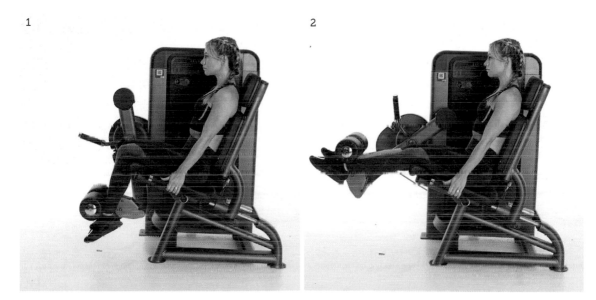

2 BULGARIAN SPLIT SQUATS ON SMITH MACHINE
x 4 sets x 12 reps on each leg

You may not need to add a weight for this exercise as it is challenging unweighted. If you would like to try a weight, make sure it is the same on each side of the bar. »> Place the bench about 0.5m behind you, so you are sandwiched between the Smith and the bench. »> Find the centre of the horizontal bar and duck underneath it, so the bar is resting across your shoulders. »> Place one foot up on the bench behind you, resting top down. Make sure the toes of your standing foot are pointing forwards. »> Take hold of the bar either side of your shoulders and unhook the bar from the machine – keep it unhooked using your grip. »> Standing up straight and bending only at the hip and knee, come down into a low squat before pushing back up through your heel to a standing position. Take a breath and repeat on the other leg. Repeat for the full amount of sets and reps.

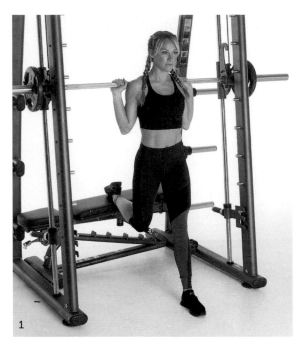

1

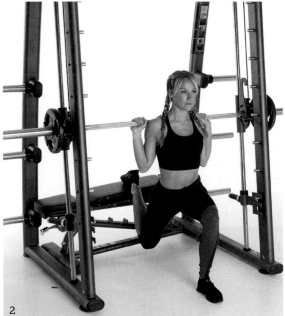

2

3 ROMANIAN DEADLIFTS WITH OLYMPIC BAR
x 4 sets x 12 reps

Place the Olympic bar in front of your feet. If you are new to lifting, you may not need to add a weight for this exercise as the Olympic bar is already weighted. If you would like to try a weight, make sure it is the same on each side of the bar. Also make sure you use bar clips whenever you use the Olympic bar, placed either side of the weight plate. »> Stand up straight with your feet hip-width apart and your toes pointing forwards. »> Keeping your back straight and bending only at the hips and knees, crouch down so your hands are now able to grasp the bar. Grasp it either side of your legs, placing one hand in an overhand grip, the other in an underhand grip (whichever hand is more comfortable is fine). »> Once you have a good grip on the bar, stand up straight, pushing down through your heels as you do so. As you come into a full standing position, squeeze your buttocks at the top of the movement. »> Pull your shoulders back, like there is a corset between your shoulder blades, and *keep them back* during this exercise. Engage your core and make sure to keep your entire core and back position solid throughout. »> Keeping the bar against your legs, slowly allow it to pull you down from the hips as far as your hamstrings will allow – sticking your bottom out as you go. »> Take a breath and return to your starting position. Repeat the lift for the full amount of sets and reps.

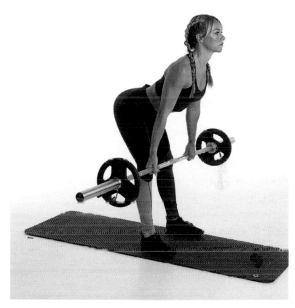

1

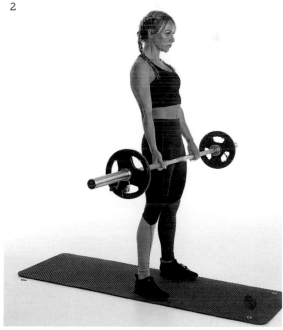

2

LOWER BODY MONDAY + THURSDAY

4 LEG PRESS ON MACHINE x 4 sets x 12 reps

Make sure the weight is the same on each side of the bar. »» Sit down on the machine and place your feet hip-width apart on the plate in front of you (or slightly further apart if that is more comfortable). Keep your toes pointing upwards, or slightly outwards, whichever you prefer. »» Pushing through the flats of your feet, slowly and gently push the plate away from your lower body. »» Using the handles either side of the chair, move the ledge that is holding the plate in place. Once the plate is free, slowly let it come towards you until you cannot retreat your legs any further. »» At this point, slowly push the plate away until you are back in your starting position. Never lock your knees out, you should always keep a slight bend in them when performing any lower body lift. »» Take a breath and repeat this movement for the full amount of sets and reps.

1
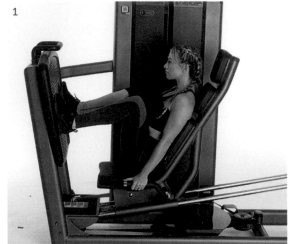

2
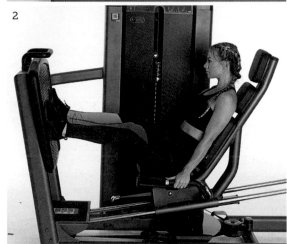

5 HIP THRUSTS ON SMITH MACHINE x 4 sets x 12 reps

If you are new to lifting, you may not need to add a weight as this exercise is challenging unweighted. If you would like to try a weight, make sure it is the same on each side of the bar. »» Place a bench about 0.5m behind you, so you are sandwiched between the Smith and the bench. »» Lower the bar so it is about 30cm off the ground. »» Sit down between the bar and the bench, facing the bar and resting your upper back and shoulder blades on the edge of the bench. Place a bar pad (a black, cushioned tube) around the centre of the horizontal bar. Place your feet hip-width apart and keep your toes pointing forwards or slightly outwards. Place your hips underneath the cushion and your hands either side of your hips. »» Unhook the bar from the machine – keep it unhooked using your grip – and thrust up into the air, through your glutes, squeezing them tight at the top of the movement. Hold this position for a few seconds before coming back down until your buttocks are just above the ground. »» Take a breath and repeat the movement for the full amount of sets and reps.

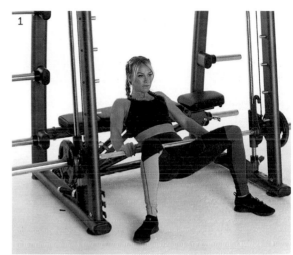

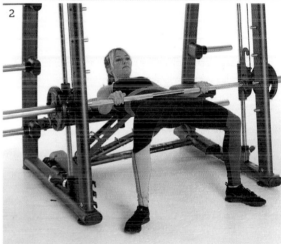

LOWER BODY MONDAY + THURSDAY

5 ABDUCTOR MACHINE x 4 sets x 12 reps

Sit on the machine and, using the prong at the side of the chair, alter the pads so that your knees are as close together as possible. »» Sit up straight and, using your knees, slowly push the pads outwards and squeeze your buttocks, engaging your glutes, as you do so (I like to do a little seated hip thrust to really engage my glutes here). »» Hold this position for a moment before slowly coming back into your starting position. »» Take a deep breath and repeat this movement for the full sets and reps.

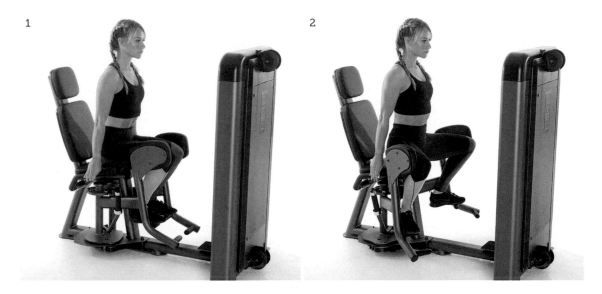

1

2

Everybody is different but, for me, the abductor machine is the most effective glute exercise. You can perform this movement sitting upright, slightly forwards or slightly back against the seat. Have a play around and see how you feel it best.

HIIT MONDAY + THURSDAY

HIIT CARDIO
ANY CARDIO MACHINE OR KETTLEBELL SWINGS: ½ MINUTE »
REST: 1½ MINUTES » REPEAT X 13 TIMES » 100% EFFORT!
TOTAL: 26 MINUTES

HIIT » KETTLEBELL SWINGS 100% EFFORT!

Stand over the kettlebell, feet slightly wider than hip-width apart. »» Squat down and grip the kettlebell with both hands. »» Pull your shoulders back, engage your core and thrust through your glutes and hips, launching the kettlebell up into the air in front of you. »» Aim to swing up to chest height, then allow the kettlebell to swing back down between your legs, keeping full control of your upper body while this happens. »» Repeat this movement fluidly and aggressively for 30 seconds before resting for 1½ minutes. Repeat 13 times.

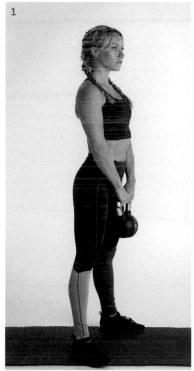
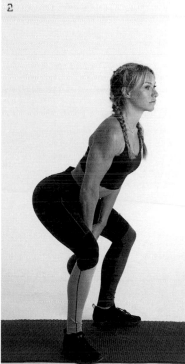
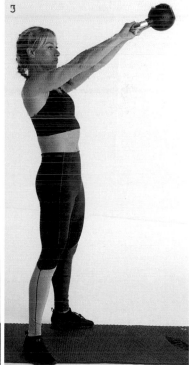

Tuesday + Saturday

WARM UP (SEE PAGES 42–51)

UPPER BODY

EXERCISES 1–6: x 4 SETS x 12 REPS

followed by

LOW–MODERATE INTENSITY CARDIO

ANY CARDIO MACHINE OR SWIMMING
FOR 30 MINUTES

COOL DOWN (SEE PAGES 42–51)

While I don't want you performing HIIT every day, I don't want you slacking during LISS or MISS cardio either. Make sure you can finish the session but, equally, I want you to push yourself for the full 30 minutes.

1 WALK OUT PUSH UPS x 1 set to exhaust

Stand up straight with your feet hip width apart. Allowing your knees to bend slightly, come down and forwards, so that your hands touch the floor, palms flat and shoulder-width apart. Crawl forwards until you are fully extended in a horizontal position. Keeping your back straight and bending only at the elbows, perform a push up. Crawl your hands back until you can stand upright again. Repeat this movement to exhaust.

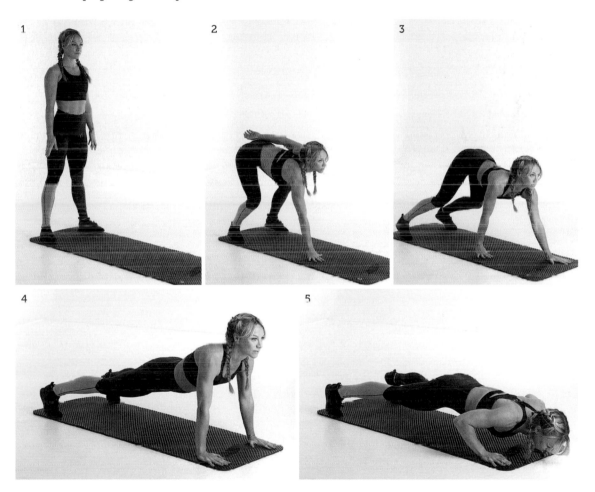

UPPER BODY TUESDAY + SATURDAY

2 CHEST PRESS ON BENCH x 4 sets x 12 reps

You will need a bench as well as dumbbells for this exercise. Make sure the dumbbell weight is the same in each hand. »» Sit on the bench with your feet flat on the floor on either side and grip the dumbbells in your hands, resting them on your thighs. »» Lie down on the bench and pull the dumbbells up so they are just above either side of your chest, making sure they are now horizontal. »» Slowly push the dumbbells up until your arms are fully extended, bringing them together at the peak of the lift so they lightly touch. »» Slowly bring the dumbbells back down to the starting position. »» Take a breath and repeat this movement for the full amount of sets and reps.

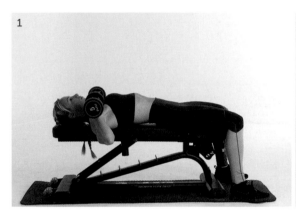
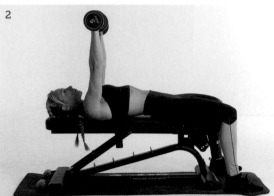

3 CHEST FLY WITH DUMBBELLS ON BENCH x 4 sets x 12 reps

You will need a bench as well as dumbbells for this exercise. Make sure the weight is the same in each hand. »» Sit on the bench with your feet flat on the floor on either side and grip the dumbbells in your hands, resting them on top of your thighs. »» Lie down on the bench. Keeping the dumbbells vertical in your grip, extend your arms out either side of your body at chest height. »» Then, as if you are hugging a beach ball and keeping a slight bend in your elbows, bring the dumbbells together above your body. »» Slowly bring the dumbbells back down to the starting position. »» Take a breath and repeat this movement for the full amount of sets and reps.

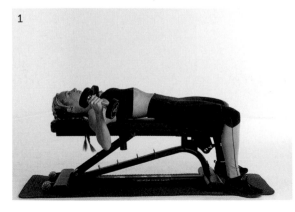
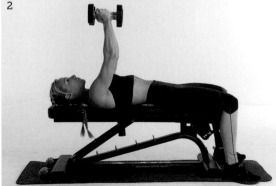

4 MOUNTAIN CLIMBERS x 1 set to exhaust

Lie on your front, feet hip-width apart, toes facing towards the floor. Place your hands by the sides of your chest, palms to the floor. Push yourself up using your hands and feet. Bring one knee up to your chest and then return it to the starting position. As you do this, switch legs. Continue this movement to exhaust.

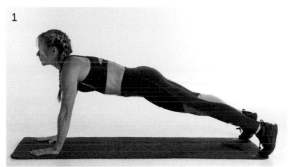

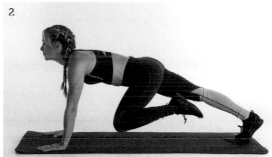

5 BICEP CURLS WITH DUMBELLS x 4 sets x 12 reps on each arm

Stand up straight with your feet hip-width apart. Grip a dumbbell in each hand and allow them to hang either side of your hips. »» Keeping your arms in tight to your sides at all times, slowly lift one dumbbell from hip height into your shoulder, twisting the dumbbell into a horizontal position as you do so. »» Slowly lower the dumbbell back down to its starting position. »» Repeat on the opposite arm. »» Continue this movement alternately for the full amount of sets and reps.

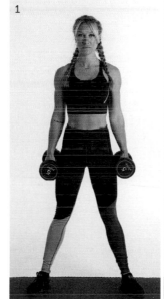

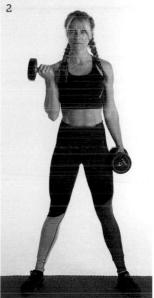

UPPER BODY TUESDAY + SATURDAY

6 TRICEP ROPE PULL DOWNS ON CABLE MACHINE
x 4 sets x 12 reps

Attach the rope pulley to the cable. Bring the cable up or down as necessary until it is above head height but within reach. »» Grip both sides of the rope with your hands, fists together and touching. »» Stand upright and engage your core. »» Using your triceps, pull the rope down until your arms are fully extended (downwards). Simultaneously, pull both sides of the rope outwards, so they end up in front of your thighs. »» Hold this extension for a second, then slowly allow the rope to travel back up above your head into your starting position. »» Take a breath and repeat this movement for the full amount of sets and reps.

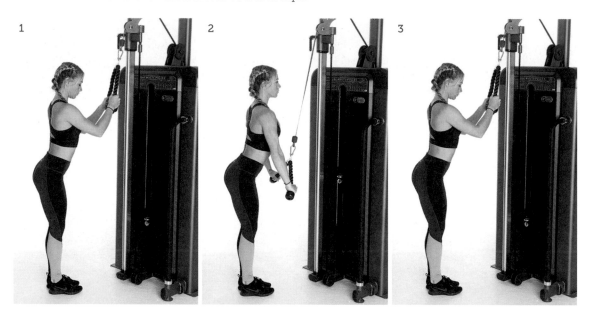

Whether you choose to use the cable machine, dumbbells or even body weight, resistance training is resistance training. If you would rather do a dip than a pull, or a lunge than a squat, that is totally fine. Just make sure you are always hitting the intended muscle and try to switch it up at least some of the time.

Wednesday + Sunday
WARM UP (SEE PAGES 42–51)
ABS
EXERCISES 1–6: x 1 SET TO EXHAUST
followed by
LOW–MODERATE INTENSITY CARDIO
ANY CARDIO MACHINE OR SWIMMING
FOR 30 MINUTES
COOL DOWN (SEE PAGES 42–51)

1 V SIT UPS WITH DUMBBELL ON MAT x 1 set to exhaust

You will need a mat for this exercise. Lie down, fully extended on the mat, gripping the weight in front of your chest, with your knees and ankles together in front of you. Extend your arms out above your head, so you are now fully stretched out, with the weight above your head. Using your arms and abdominals, slowly and gradually bring your upper body into a crunch, simultaneously lifting your legs up off the ground and into the air (your shins and the weight should meet half way). Slowly and gradually come back down into your starting position. Repeat this movement fluidly to exhaust.

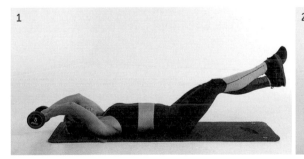
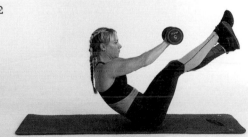

ABS WEDNESDAY + SUNDAY

2 LEG RAISES ON MAT x 1 set to exhaust

You will need a mat or a soft surface for this exercise. Lie on your back, extending your legs out fully and crossing your ankles. Keep your arms flat by your sides – feel free to hold on to the sides of the mat or on to a solid object behind your head to make this movement easier. Slowly raise your legs up into the air so they are vertical above your body, give a little upward thrust with your hips, raising your bottom off the floor, then slowly bring your legs back down to just above ground level. Repeat this movement to exhaust.

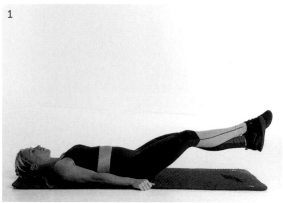

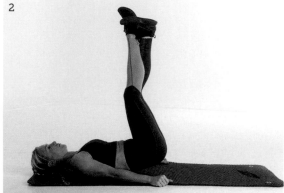

3 PLANK x 1 hold to exhaust

You may need a mat or cushion for your elbows during this exercise. Lie on your front with your feet hip-width apart, resting your toes against the top of the mat. Rest on your elbows and keep your forearms flat against the mat. Make sure your elbows are below your shoulders. Pushing against your toes and forearms, raise your body up into an elevated plank. *Do not* allow your spine to curve, either concavely or convexly – you want a straight back. Hold this position to exhaust. If you are struggling, feel free to transfer your weight from one foot to another, essentially shuffling your feet while holding the plank position.

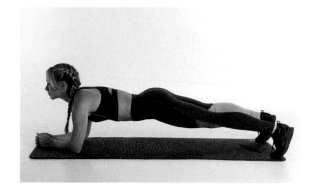

4 SIDE BENDS UNWEIGHTED x 1 set to exhaust

Stand up straight with your feet hip-width apart, your arms flat by your sides, and your fingertips pointing down towards the floor. Engage your core, tensing your mid-section as if you are about to be punched in the stomach. Slowly and in a controlled manner, bend to one side as far as your natural range will allow. Still tensing your stomach, use your core to come back up to a straight, standing position (again, do this slowly and in a controlled manner). Repeat this movement on the opposite side. Continue to perform alternately to exhaust.

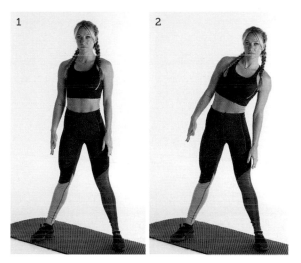

5 HEEL TAPS x 1 set to exhaust

You may need a mat or a soft surface to cushion your back for this exercise. Lie on your back with your knees bent and your feet on the floor hip-width apart. Doing a very slight abdominal crunch so your upper back is slightly raised off the ground, stretch out your hands and move slowly to your right and left, repetitively, touching the outsides of your feet as you do so. Continue to perform this exercise to exhaust.

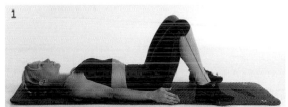

6 RUSSIAN TWISTS WITH WEIGHT PLATE x 1 set to exhaust

You will need a mat for this exercise. Sit upright on the mat, knees slightly bent and your ankles crossed in front of you. Raise your ankles up off the ground by 5cm or so and hold the weight out in front of your stomach. Slowly twist your abdominals and upper body to one side, allowing the weight to touch the mat beside your hips. Bring the weight back to the centre and repeat this move on the other side. Repeat this movement fluidly to exhaust.

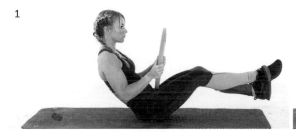
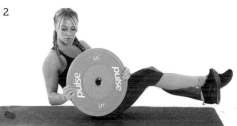

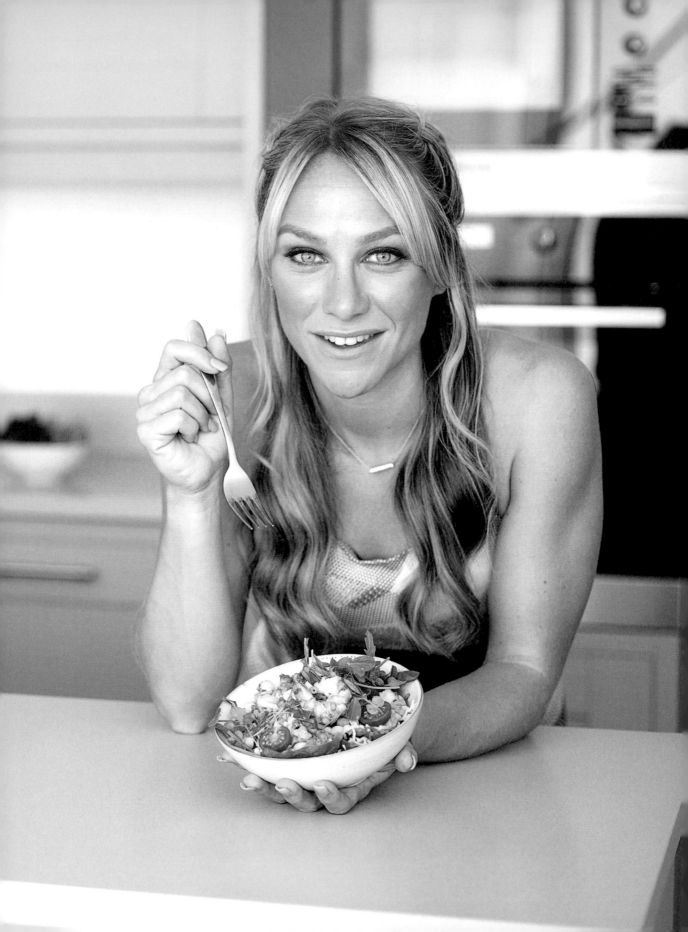

RECIPES

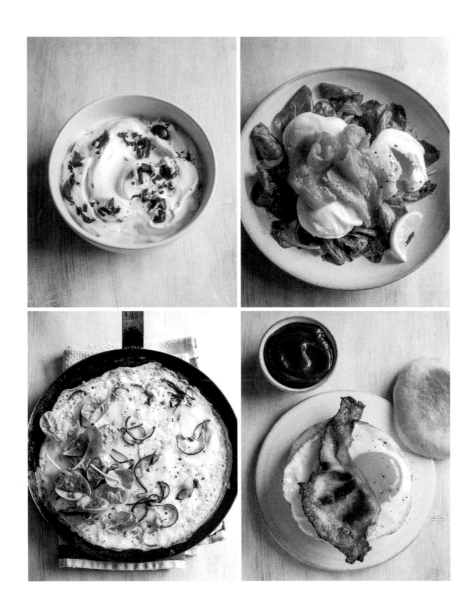

BREAKFASTS

Chocolate Chip Overnight Oats

I started making this recently and it is delicious!

SERVES 1

30g plain oats (typically 1 sachet or 3 level tbsp)

1 scoop whey protein powder (typically 25–30g)

2 squares 90% dark chocolate (typically 25g), broken into little pieces

approx. 200ml any milk option (see The Food Bible)

1 tsp Sweet Freedom Choc Shot (optional

1 Mix the oats, protein powder and chocolate pieces together in a small bowl.

2 Gradually pour milk over the mixture, stirring all the time, until the ingredients are combined and slightly submerged.

3 Drizzle with Sweet Freedom Choc Shot, if using, then refrigerate overnight (or for no less than 4 hours).

HIGH
CARB

Crunchy Granola Bowl

I love granola but it's so high in calories that you can't have much of it on a diet. This is a great way to satiate granola cravings!

SERVES 1

1 small handful plain granola (approx. 30g)

1 small pot 0% Greek yoghurt (typically 170g)

1 level tbsp any crunchy nut butter (approx. 15g)

1 tsp MYPROTEIN Sugar-free Syrup (optional)

1 Combine the granola, yoghurt and nut butter together in a bowl.

2 Drizzle with MYPROTEIN Sugar-free Syrup, if using, and serve.

Breakfast Shake

This is perfect for those of you who love fruit smoothies!

SERVES 1

1 medium banana

½ small pot 0% Greek yoghurt (typically 85g)

1 heaped tbsp desiccated coconut (approx. 25g)

500ml unsweetened coconut milk

1 Whizz all the ingredients together in a blender until you reach the desired consistency.

2 Pour into a glass to serve.

Black Forest Bowl

This idea came to me recently so I made it for
my partner and he loved it!

SERVES 1

¼ × 400g tin pitted black
cherries

1 small pot 0% Greek yoghurt
(typically 170g)

2 squares 90% dark chocolate
(typically 25g), broken into
little pieces

1 tsp Sweet Freedom Choc
Shot (optional)

1 Combine the cherries, yoghurt and chocolate
pieces together in a bowl.

2 Drizzle with Sweet Freedom Choc Shot,
if using, and serve.

Peanut Butter Proats

This is an old staple of mine...

SERVES 1

30g plain oats (typically
1 sachet or 3 level tbsp)

1 scoop whey protein powder
(typically 25–30g)

1 level tbsp peanut butter
(approx. 15g)

1 tsp MYPROTEIN Sugar-free
Syrup (optional)

1 Mix the oats, protein powder and peanut
butter together in a bowl.

2 Gradually pour boiling water over the
mixture, stirring all the time, until you reach
the desired consistency.

3 Drizzle with MYPROTEIN Sugar-free Syrup,
if using, and serve.

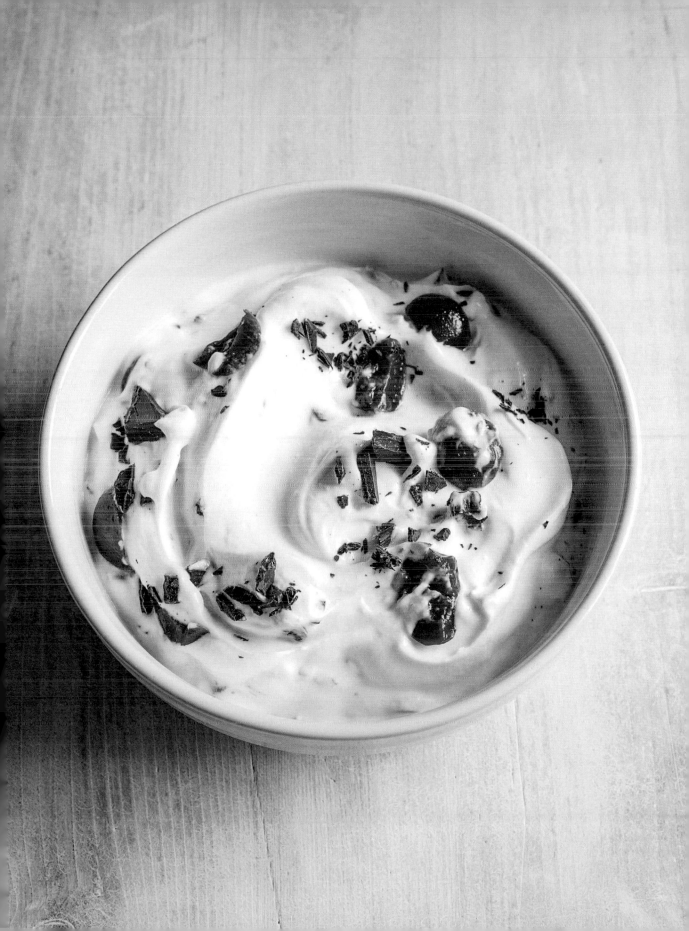

**HIGH
CARB**

The Muffin Man

There's something heartwarming about
a runny egg in an English muffin.

SERVES 1

2 knife smears butter
   (typically 10g)
1 English muffin, halved
   and toasted
1 spray Fry Light cooking
   spray (optional)
1 slice bacon
1 whole egg
1 tsp Heinz Reduced Salt and
   Sugar Ketchup (optional)

1 Butter the toasted muffin, then place it to
one side.

2 Spray a small frying pan with Fry Light,
if using, and place over a high heat. Add
the bacon and fry to the desired crispiness.

3 Using the same pan, crack in the egg and
fry sunny side up.

4 Carefully place the egg on one half of the
muffin then top with the bacon, drizzle with
ketchup, if using, and sandwich with the
other muffin half.

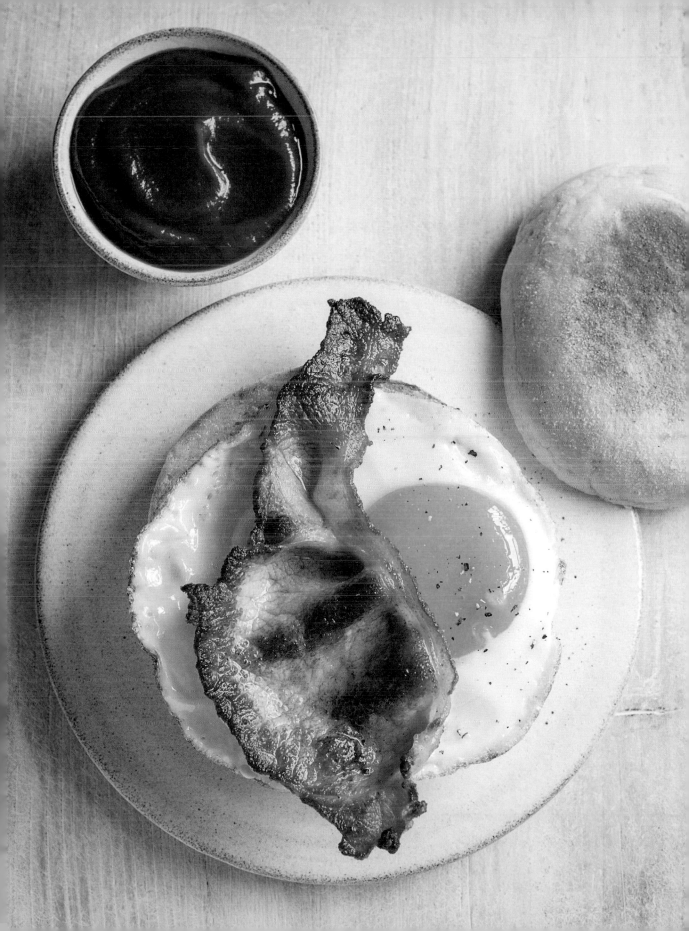

Breakfast Burrito

Still my all-time favourite meal, any time of the day!

SERVES 1

1 spray Fry Light cooking
    spray (optional)
1 slice bacon (any)
1 small tortilla wrap (any)
1 whole egg
½ avocado, diced
½ tomato, diced
1 tsp Tabasco (optional)

1 Place a frying pan over a high heat and spray with Fry Light, if using.

2 Add the bacon and fry to the desired crispness.

3 Place the tortilla on a serving plate, and top with the bacon.

4 Using the same pan, crack in the egg and cook, stirring, until scrambled. Remove from the pan and place on top of bacon in the middle of the tortilla.

5 Finally, add the avocado and tomato to the tortilla and drizzle with Tabasco, if using.

6 Fold the bottom of the tortilla up to cover the bottom of the filling. Fold one side of the tortilla over the filling, then continue to roll it over to the other side until wrapped, then serve.

Mini Pitta Party

This may be small but the carb and fat combo make it filling!

SERVES 1

1 mini pitta (wholegrain)

1 level tsp butter (approx. 10g)

1 spray Fry Light cooking spray (optional)

1 slice halloumi (typically 30g)

1 slice bacon

1 whole egg

1 Toast the pitta and cut an opening in the top.

2 Butter the inside of the pitta.

3 Place a frying pan over a high heat and spray with Fry Light, if using. When the pan is hot, add the halloumi and cook for about 3 minutes on each side, until golden brown. Remove from the pan and place inside the pitta.

4 Add the bacon to the pan and cook until the desired crispness. Remove from the pan and place inside the pitta.

5 Using the same pan, crack in the egg and cook, stirring, until scrambled. Remove from the pan, place inside the pitta and serve.

Smoked Salmon Bagel Thin

An old classic and one that deserves a mention!

SERVES 1

1 plain bagel thin, halved and toasted
1 level tbsp full-fat cream cheese (approx. 30g)
4 slices smoked salmon (typically 80g)
juice of ½ lemon
rocket, to serve (optional)

1 Spread both bagel halves with cream cheese and divide the smoked salmon between them.

2 Drizzle with lemon juice and serve with rocket, if using.

Warm Winter PeanutBix

Eagle-eyed Blitzers will wonder where the protein is in this breakfast – the combination of peanut butter and wheat form a complete protein.

SERVES 1

1 level tbsp smooth peanut butter (approx. 15g)
2 Weetabix
approx. 200ml any milk option (see The Food Bible)
1 tsp Sweet Freedom Choc Shot (optional)

1 Spread the peanut butter over the Weetabix biscuits and place them in a bowl.

2 Pour the milk over the top until partially covered.

3 Place in a microwave and warm for 1 minute on a medium heat.

4 Drizzle with Sweet Freedom Choc Shot, if using, and serve.

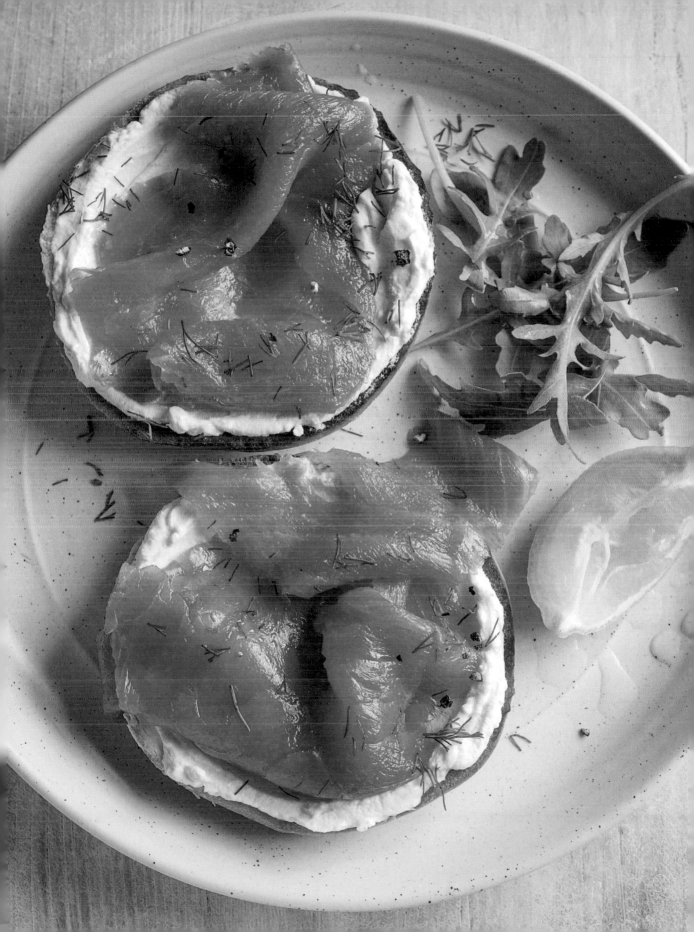

Chocolate Almond Protein Cake

People really struggled to make the protein pancakes in the first book, so here is a *much* quicker and easier option!

SERVES 1

1 scoop protein powder (typically 25–30g)

approx. 100ml any milk option (see The Food Bible)

1 level tbsp almond butter (approx. 15g)

1 square 99% dark chocolate (typically 10–15g), grated

1 Mix the protein powder and milk in a small bowl until it is a thick batter (similar to the consistency of very thick custard).

2 Dot with the almond butter and sprinkle with the chocolate.

3 Microwave on high for 2 minutes.

4 Leave to cool for 1 minute before eating.

LOW
CARB

Coconut Protein Shake

This is simple and perfect for those on the go!

SERVES 1

1 scoop protein powder
(typically 25–30g)
approx. 500ml unsweetened
coconut milk
1 heaped tbsp desiccated
coconut (approx. 25g)

1 Shake or blend all the ingredients together
until you reach the desired consistency.

2 Pour into a tall glass and serve.

Sweet Almond Whip

This is a nice alternative for those who miss their granola!

SERVES 1

1 small pot 0% Greek yoghurt
(typically 170g)
1 level tbsp almond butter
(approx. 15g)
1 small handful almonds
(approx. 20g)
1 tsp any MYPROTEIN
Sugar-free Syrup (optional)

1 Mix all the ingredients together in a bowl.

2 Drizzle with MYPROTEIN Sugar-free Syrup,
if using, and serve.

Cheese and Onion Omelette

It's an oldie, but it's a goodie!

SERVES 1

1 level tsp butter (approx. 10g)

½ small red onion (typically 50g), thinly sliced

2 whole eggs

1 small handful grated Cheddar (approx. 30g)

1 large handful spinach and/or rocket

1 Melt the butter in a frying pan over a medium heat, add the onion and cook for 4–5 minutes to soften.

2 Meanwhile, crack the eggs into a small bowl and whisk with a fork. Season with a little salt and pepper, then pour into the pan with the onion and swirl the pan clockwise to level out.

3 Sprinkle the Cheddar over the top and continue to cook until the omelette has reached your desired consistency.

4 Place a bed of spinach and/or rocket on your serving plate, fold one half of the omelette over the other with a spatula and place on top of the rocket to serve.

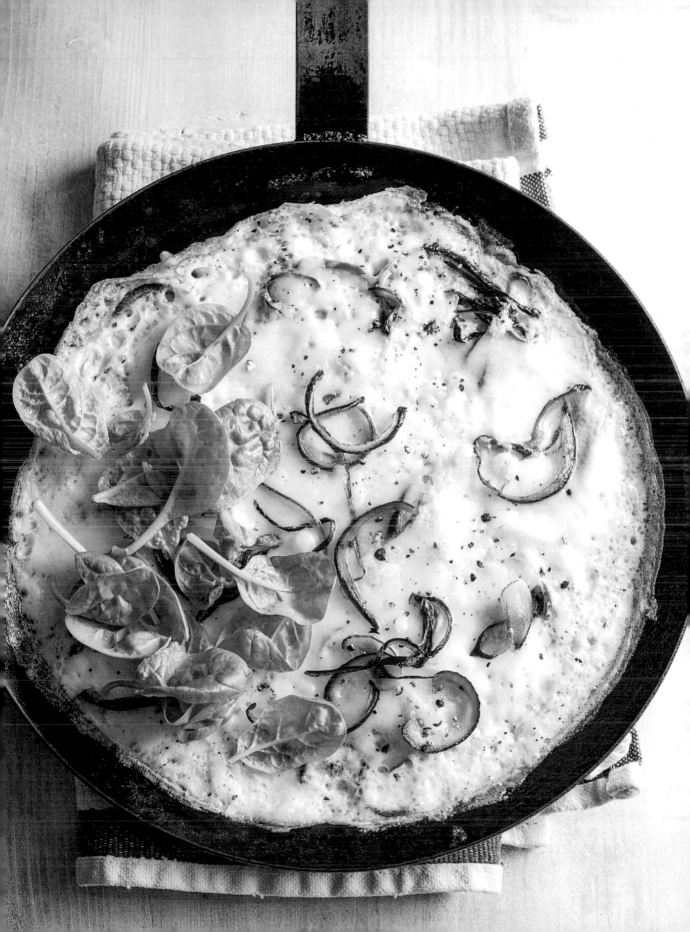

Lo-Dough Breakfast Burrito

I don't want to include too many 'speciality' foods in these recipes, but, for me, Lo-Dough is a low-carb dietary saviour and it deserves a mention (you can find it online).

SERVES 1

1 piece Lo-Dough
1 spray Fry Light cooking spray (optional)
1 slice bacon
2 whole eggs
½ tomato, diced
½ avocado, diced
1 tsp Tabasco (optional)

1 Place the Lo-Dough in a frying pan over a low heat to warm.

2 Meanwhile, place a separate frying pan over a high heat and spray with Fry Light, if using. Add the bacon and fry to the desired crispness.

3 Remove the bacon from the pan and place in the centre of the Lo-Dough.

4 Using the bacon pan, crack in the egg and cook, stirring, until scrambled, then place on top of the bacon.

5 Top with the tomato and avocado and drizzle with Tabasco, if using.

6 Fold the bottom of the dough over the bottom of the filling, then hold the bottom in place as you roll one side of the dough over the filling until you have a wrap.

Bacon Dippy Eggs

I saw this on Instagram last year and started
making it for my partner as a snack!

SERVES 1

4 slices bacon
4 asparagus spears
2 whole eggs

1 Preheat the oven to 200°C/fan 180°C.

2 Stretch out each slice of bacon with the
back of a knife to lengthen, then wrap each
one around an asparagus spear.

3 Place the wrapped spears on a baking sheet
and bake for 20 minutes, or until the bacon
is crisp.

4 Meanwhile, boil the eggs until soft boiled.

5 Serve the asparagus and bacon with the
soft-boiled eggs and dip them in like toast
soldiers.

Smoked Salmon Eggs Florentine

This breakfast both looks and tastes truly beautiful!

SERVES 1

generous dash malt vinegar
4 whole eggs
1 level tsp butter (approx. 10g)
1 large handful spinach
2 slices smoked salmon
   (typically 40g)
½ lemon

1 Bring a large pan of water to the boil, then reduce to a simmer. Add the vinegar, then stir the water clockwise.

2 Crack the eggs into the centre of the swirling water one at a time and leave to simmer for approximately 3 minutes.

3 Meanwhile, melt the butter in a large pan over a medium heat, add the spinach and leave to wilt.

4 Remove the spinach from the pan and spread evenly over a plate.

5 Remove the eggs from their pan using a slotted spoon and place on top of the spinach.

6 Place the smoked salmon over the eggs, drizzle with lemon juice and serve.

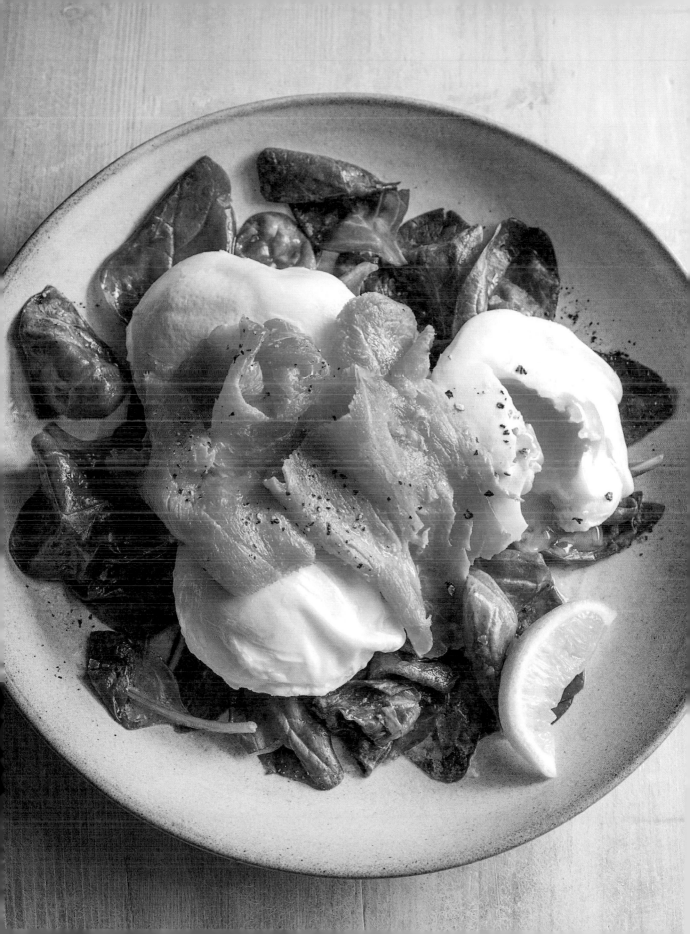

Sausage and Egg Patties

For those of you who love a naughty brekkers!

SERVES 1

2 small pork sausages
2 sprays Fry Light cooking
   spray (optional)
2 whole eggs
1 tsp Heinz Reduced Salt and
   Sugar Ketchup (optional)

1 Remove the sausage meat from the skins and use the palms of your hands to mould it into 2 flat discs.

2 Place a frying pan over a medium–high heat and spray with Fry Light, if using. Add the patties and cook for approximately 4–5 minutes on each side.

3 Remove them from the pan and place in the centre of your serving plate.

4 Spray more Fry Light into the pan, if using, and crack in the eggs. Fry them sunny side up for about 5 minutes, depending on how you like your eggs, then place them on top of the sausage patties.

5 Season, drizzle with ketchup, if using, and serve.

LOW
CARB

Turkey Bacon Rolls

This is a sort of breakfast salad I had at a café
recently and it blew my mind!

SERVES 1

2 slices halloumi
(typically 60g)
4 slices turkey bacon
1 large handful spinach and/
or rocket

1 Preheat the oven to 200°C/fan 180°C.

2 Quarter both halloumi slices to make
8 thick slabs.

3 Stretch each of the 4 turkey bacon rashers
out with the back of a knife, then cut each
rasher in half to make 8 slices.

4 Wrap each slice of turkey bacon around
a chunk of halloumi and place them on a
baking sheet.

5 Bake for 20 minutes, or until the bacon
is brown and beginning to crisp.

6 Place a generous bed of spinach and/or
rocket on your serving plate, top with the
halloumi rolls and serve.

Turkish Eggs

My new favourite – this is packed full of flavour
and incredibly filling.

SERVES 1

1 level tsp butter (approx. 10g)
½ small white onion
   (typically 50g), peeled
   and diced
1 large handful spinach
½ × 400g tin chopped
   tomatoes
3 whole eggs

1 Melt the butter in a small frying pan over
a medium heat and add the onion. Cook for
4–5 minutes to soften, then add the spinach
and allow to wilt.

2 Add the chopped tomatoes, season well
with salt and pepper and leave to simmer
for 5–10 minutes.

3 Using the back of a spoon, create 3 small
dents in the mixture and crack an egg into
each one. Cover the pan with a lid, reduce
the temperature to low and leave the eggs
to cook for 5–10 minutes, depending on
how soft you want the yolks.

4 Remove from the heat and serve.

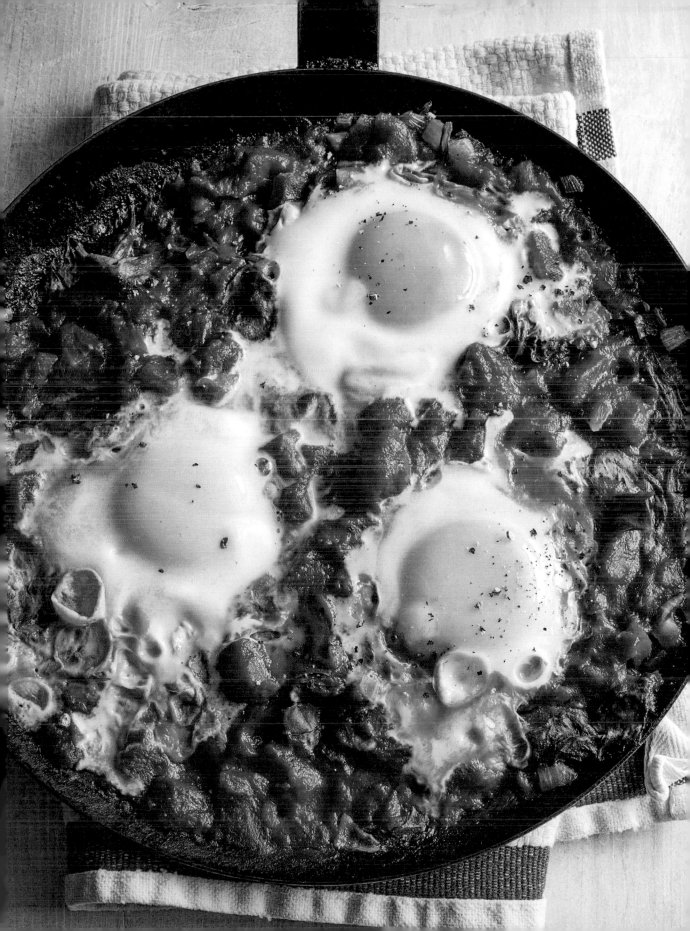

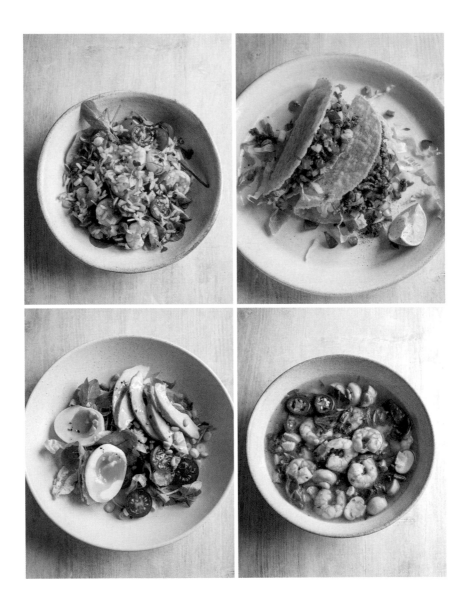

LUNCHES
AND
DINNERS

TLT

A healthy take on a BLT!

SERVES 1

1 spray Fry Light cooking spray (optional)
2 slices turkey bacon
2 small slices bread (wholegrain)
2 knife smears butter (typically 10g)
½ tomato, sliced into 4
4 small lettuce leaves
1 tsp Heinz Reduced Salt and Sugar Ketchup (optional)

1 Place a small frying pan over a high heat and spray with Fry Light, if using.

2 Add the turkey bacon and cook for 4–5 minutes, or until you reach the desired crispness.

3 Meanwhile, butter the bread (or toast, if you prefer) and place 2 lettuce leaves on top of each piece of bread. Top with the tomato.

4 Remove the bacon from the pan and place it in the centre of the sandwich.

5 Drizzle with ketchup, if using, and sandwich the halves together to serve.

Chicken Pesto Penne Pasta

This is an old-school favourite of mine.

SERVES 1

1 small chicken breast
(typically 125g)
40g penne pasta
(uncooked weight)
2 level tbsp any pesto
(approx. 30g)
1 large handful rocket

1 Preheat the oven to 200°C/fan 180°C.

2 Season the chicken breast and bake uncovered in the oven for 20–30 minutes, or until the juices run clear.

3 Meanwhile, cook the pasta according to the packet instructions.

4 Drain the penne and return it to the pan.

5 Remove the chicken from the oven and, using 2 forks, shred the meat, then add it to the pasta.

6 Stir in the pesto, season with salt and pepper and serve on a bed of rocket.

Prawn Rice Salad

This is perfect for when you're craving something healthy, clean and green!

SERVES 1

35g wholegrain or long grain rice (uncooked weight)

2 tsp olive oil

1 tsp chopped garlic

1 small packet raw prawns (typically 150g)

1 large handful spinach and/or rocket and/or lettuce leaves

5 cherry tomatoes, halved

1 spring onion, thinly sliced

juice of ½ lemon

1 Cook the rice according to the packet instructions and set aside.

2 Drizzle 1 teaspoon of the olive oil into a frying pan and place over a medium–high heat. Add the chopped garlic and allow to sizzle. Tip in the prawns and start to cook.

3 Before the prawns are completely pink, add the rice, season with salt and pepper and toss everything together.

4 Place the spinach or salad leaves, tomatoes and spring onion in a large salad bowl. Once the prawns are cooked through, tip in the prawn and rice mixture and combine.

5 Drizzle with lemon juice and the remaining olive oil, season again and serve.

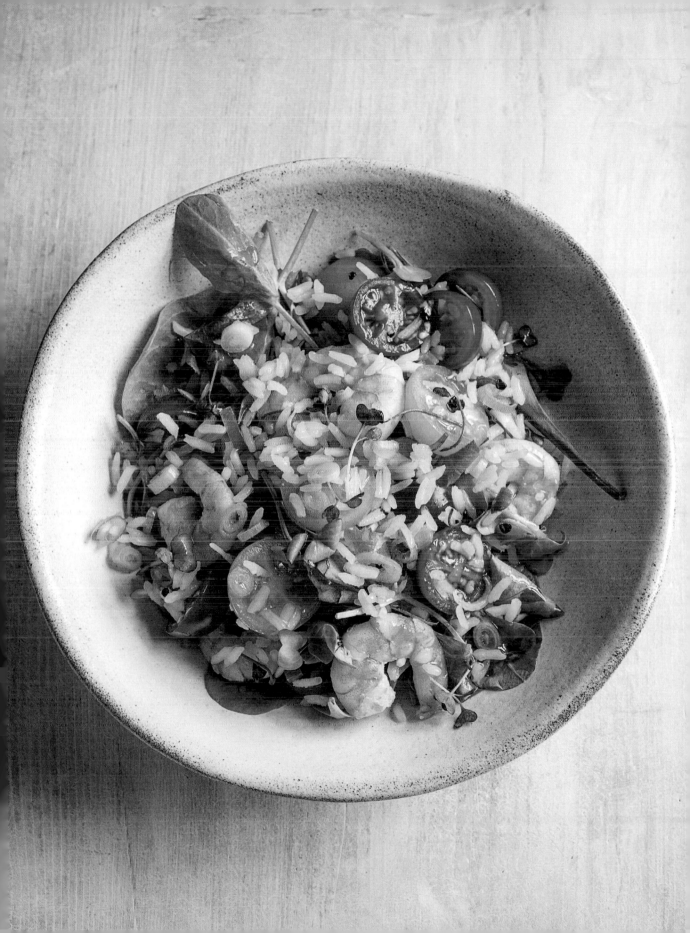

HIGH CARB

Tuna Mayo Spud

For when you're tired and hungry and you need some comfort!

SERVES 1

1 small baking potato
   (typically 150g cooked
   weight)
1 small tin tuna
   (60g drained weight)
1 level tsp mayonnaise
1 level tsp butter (approx. 10g)
1 spring onion, finely sliced
1 large handful rocket

1 Preheat the oven to 200°C/fan 180°C.

2 Rinse, dry and score the potato with a crisscross. Season well with salt and pepper, then place in the centre of the oven and bake for roughly 1 hour, or until golden brown on the outside and soft to the touch.

3 Meanwhile, mix the tuna and mayonnaise together in a small bowl.

4 Remove the potato from the oven, cut open and add the butter, using the back of a fork to mash it in.

5 Season the potato with salt and pepper, add the tuna mayo filling and sprinkle with the spring onion.

6 Serve with the rocket alongside.

Prawn and Feta Couscous

This is very filling, very tangy and very tasty!

SERVES 1

35g couscous
   (uncooked weight)
1 spray Fry Light cooking
   spray (optional)
1 small packet raw prawns
   (typically 150g)
1 small handful crumbled
   feta (approx. 40g)
1 large handful rocket
juice of ½ lemon

1 Cook the couscous according to the packet instructions.

2 Meanwhile, place a frying pan over a medium-high heat and spray with Fry Light, if using.

3 Add the prawns, season well, and toss for 2–3 minutes, or until pink.

4 Add the couscous and mix well.

5 Stir in the feta and rocket, squeeze lemon over the mixture, season and serve.

Turkey Burger

The lean burger option! You could add a pinch of dried thyme or a few chopped fresh thyme leaves when you season the mince, if you like.

SERVES 1

100g turkey breast mince
1 whole egg
1 small red onion, peeled
    and ½ diced and ½ sliced
your choice of herbs/
    spices/seasoning
1 spray Fry Light cooking
    spray (optional)
1 small bread roll (any),
    halved
1 lettuce leaf
½ small tomato, sliced
1 pickle, sliced
1 tsp Heinz Reduced Salt and
    Sugar Ketchup (optional)

1 Place the mince, egg, diced onion and seasoning together in a small bowl and mix well to combine. Mould and flatten into a burger.

2 Place a frying pan over a medium heat and spray with Fry Light, if using. Add the burger and cook for 5 minutes on each side, or until cook through.

3 Meanwhile, place the bun face down in the pan with the burger until lightly toasted.

4 Remove the bun from the pan and place on a plate. Build the burger by placing the turkey on top of the bun, then the lettuce, sliced tomato, sliced onion and pickle. Drizzle with ketchup, if using, to serve.

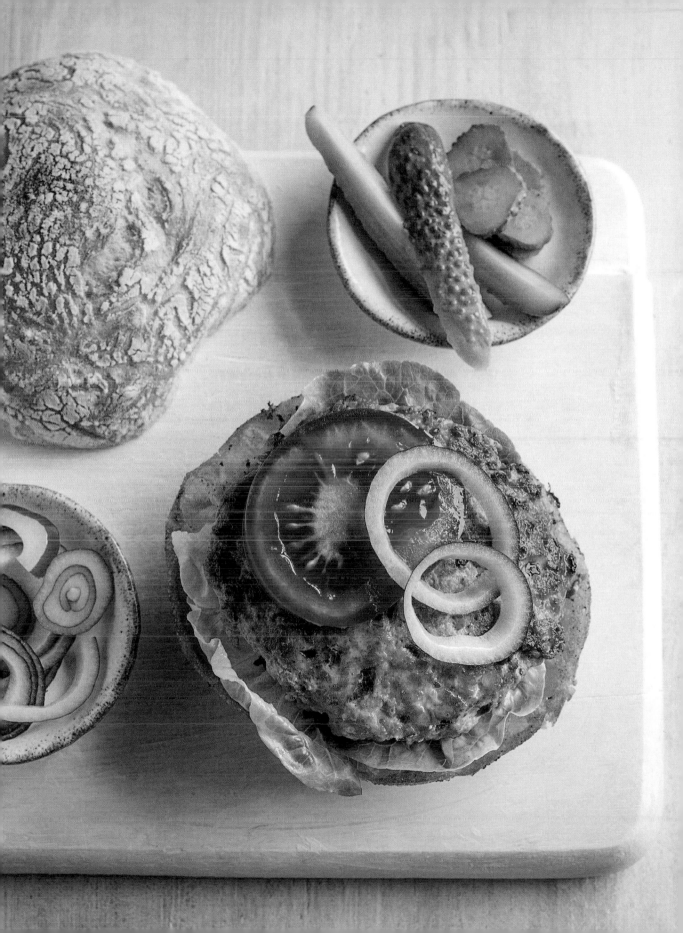

Tortilla Pizza

The healthier way to enjoy a pizza!

SERVES 1

1 plain, small tortilla wrap
   (typically 40g)

2 level tbsp passata
   (approx. 30g)

2 chicken sausages (typically
   34g each), finely sliced
   (Heck Chicken Chipolatas
   are my favourite)

½ small red onion, peeled
   and finely sliced

½ jalapeño pepper, sliced

1 small handful grated
   Cheddar (approx. 30g)

1 Preheat the oven to 200°C/fan 180°C.

2 Place the tortilla in the middle of a baking tray and spoon the passata into the middle, spreading it outwards and evenly towards the edges.

3 Scatter over the sausage slices, red onion and jalapeño, then sprinkle with the cheese.

4 Bake in the oven for 10 minutes, or until your desired crispiness.

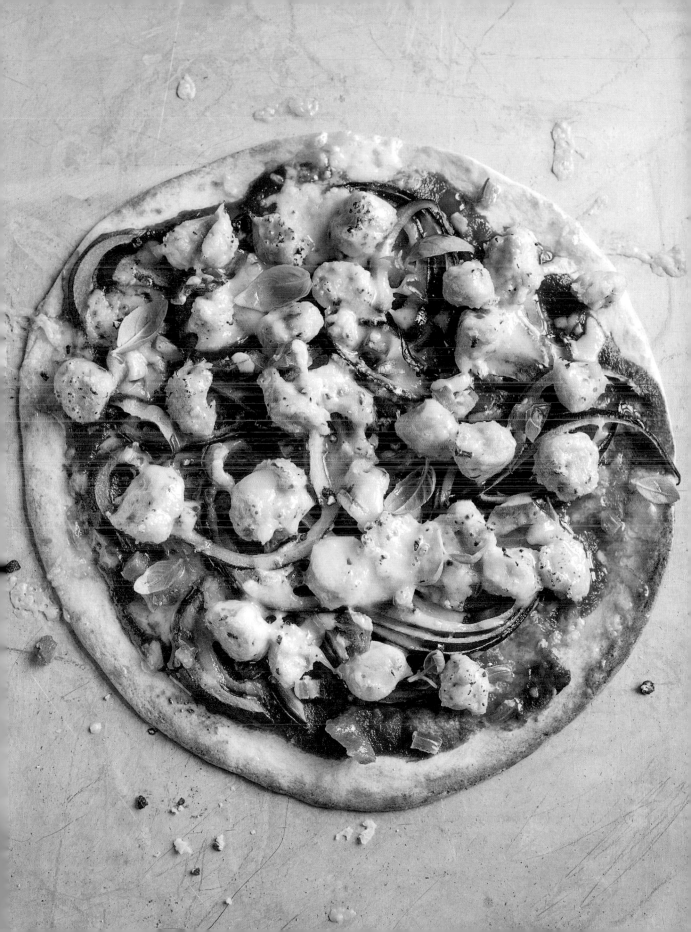

Meat and Two Veg

This is a great option when you're in need of filling up!

SERVES 1

1 small fillet steak
(typically 200g)

1 small head broccoli
(typically 200g), broken
into florets

2 small new potatoes
(typically 100g cooked
weight)

1 spray Fry Light cooking
spray (optional)

1 level tsp butter (approx. 10g)

1 tsp Heinz Reduced Salt and
Sugar Ketchup (optional)

1 Allow the steak to come up to room temperature and bring a large pan of salted water to the boil.

2 Add the broccoli and new potatoes to the pan and leave to simmer for 20–30 minutes.

3 Before the vegetables are fully cooked, season the steak on each side with salt and pepper and place a small frying pan over a high heat. Spray with Fry Light, if using, then add the steak. Sear on each side for 1 minute, or until cooked to your liking.

4 Remove from the heat and place on a plate to rest.

5 Drain the broccoli and potatoes and return them to the pan. Season well with salt and pepper, then lazily mash so that big chunks remain.

6 Add the butter to the mixture and stir well.

7 Spoon the broccoli and potatoes into the centre of a plate, top with the steak and drizzle with ketchup, if using, to serve.

HIGH
CARB

Sausage and Mash

An old classic that doesn't have to go anywhere just because you're dieting.

SERVES 1

1 small baking potato (typically 150g cooked weight), peeled and quartered

2 pork chipolatas (typically 60g)

1 level tsp butter (approx. 10g)

1 tsp Heinz Reduced Salt and Sugar Ketchup (optional)

1 Preheat the grill to high.

2 Bring a small pan of salted water to the boil and add the potato. Simmer for 20–30 minutes, or until soft when poked with a kitchen knife.

3 Meanwhile, pierce the sausages with a fork and grill for 10–15 minutes, turning occasionally, or until cooked through.

4 Drain the potato and return to the pan. Season well with salt and pepper, add the butter and mash.

5 Spoon the potato into the centre of a plate and place the chipolatas on top.

6 Drizzle with ketchup, if using, to serve.

Spicy Beef Tacos

Yup, you can eat tacos and lose weight – you just have to make them the right way! You could try adding a pinch of smoked paprika and another of chilli powder with the mince for added spice.

SERVES 1

1 spray Fry Light cooking
   spray (optional)
100g 5% beef mince
any herbs/spices/hot sauce
   desired
½ tomato, diced
½ white onion, peeled
   and diced
½ jalapeño pepper, diced
juice of ½ lime
2 taco shells
1 large handful shredded
   lettuce

1 Place a small frying pan over a medium–high heat and spray with Fry Light, if using.

2 Add the mince and cook for about 7–10 minutes, until brown. Season with salt and pepper to taste.

3 Meanwhile, place the tomato, onion and jalapeño in a small bowl and mix together with the lime juice.

4 Stuff each taco with a little lettuce, divide the mince between the two shells, then top with the salsa and serve.

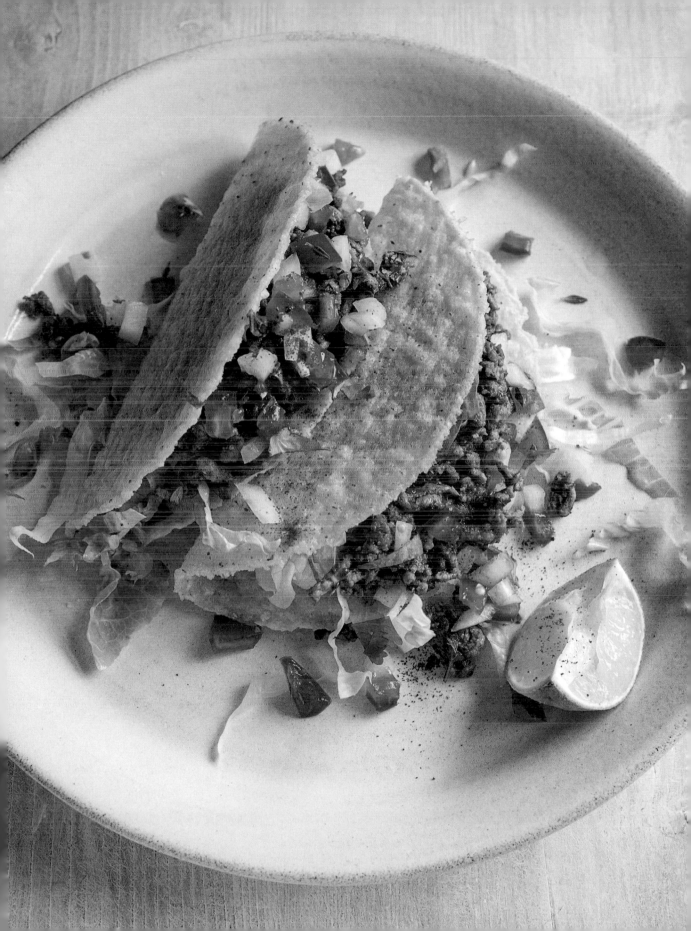

Lo-Dough Pizza

Lo-Dough is an ideal substitute for a high-carb wrap or a pizza base.

SERVES 1

1 piece Lo-Dough

2 level tbsp passata
(approx. 30g)

2 chicken sausages (typically
34g each), finely sliced
(Heck Chicken Chipolatas
are my favourite)

½ small red onion, peeled
and finely sliced

½ jalapeño pepper, finely
sliced

1 small handful grated
Cheddar (approx. 30g)

1 tsp chilli oil

1 Preheat oven to 200°C/fan 180°C.

2 Place the Lo-Dough in the middle of a
baking tray and spoon the passata into the
middle. Spread it outwards and evenly
towards the edges.

3 Arrange the sausages, onion and jalapeño
evenly around the pizza base. Sprinkle the
Cheddar over the top and bake in the oven
for 10 minutes, or until the pizza has reached
your desired crispiness.

4 Remove the pizza from the oven, cut into
quarters and serve with the chilli oil in a small
bowl alongside. Dip in and enjoy!

Meat and Three Veg

The low-carb version of the spud-centred dish!

SERVES 1

1 small fillet steak
   (typically 200g)
1 small head broccoli
   (typically 200g), broken
   into florets
1 spray Fry Light cooking
   spray (optional)
1 portobello mushroom
½ large tomato
1 level tsp butter (approx. 10g)
1 tsp Heinz Reduced Salt and
   Sugar Ketchup (optional)

1 Allow the steak to come up to room temperature and bring a large pan of salted water to the boil.

2 Add the broccoli to the pan and simmer for 20–30 minutes, until very tender.

3 Meanwhile, place a small frying pan over a high heat and spray with Fry Light, if using.

4 Season the steak on each side with salt and pepper and add to the pan with the mushroom and tomato. Sear the steak on each side for 1 minute, or until cooked to your liking.

5 Drain the broccoli and return it to the pan with the butter. Season well with salt and pepper and mash.

6 Spoon the broccoli into the centre of a serving plate and place the steak and vegetables on top.

7 Drizzle with ketchup, if using, to serve.

My Big Fat Salad

This is a hearty salad full of great fats and great greens!

SERVES 1

2 whole eggs
1 large handful spinach
   and/or rocket and/
   or lettuce leaves
5 cherry tomatoes, halved
1 spring onion,
   finely chopped
½ avocado, sliced
1 level tbsp pine nuts
   (approx. 15g)
1 tsp olive oil

1 Bring a pan of water to the boil and cook the eggs in their shells for 5–10 minutes, depending on how soft you like the yolks.

2 Meanwhile, build the salad in a large serving bowl. Place the salad leaves inside, then top with the tomatoes, spring onion, avocado and pine nuts.

3 Drain the eggs and place them under cold running water. Shell and halve them, then add to the salad bowl.

4 Season well with salt and pepper, drizzle with olive oil and serve.

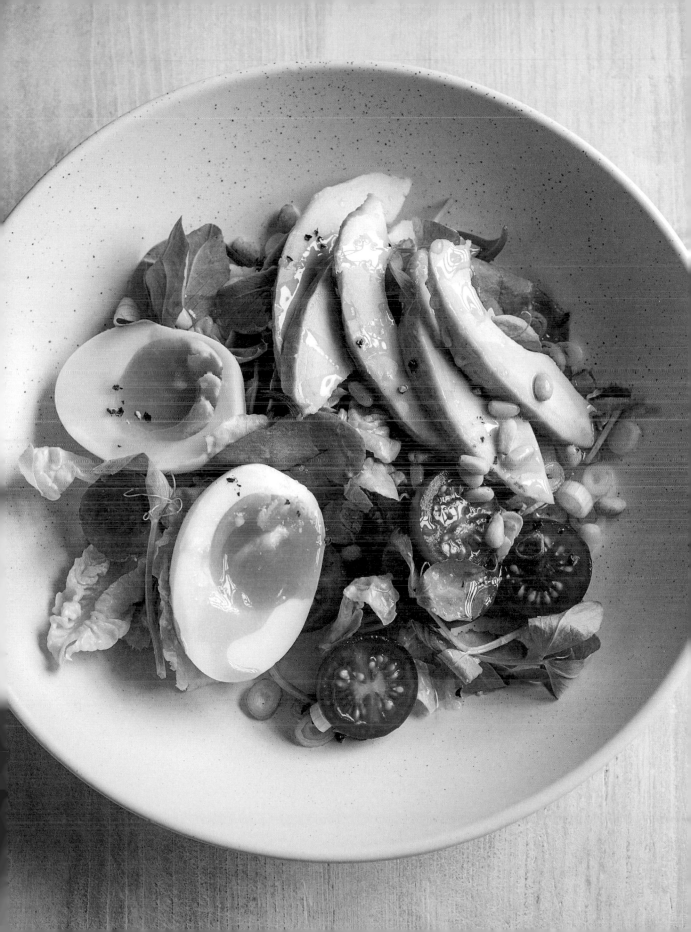

Cheesy Chicken and Cauliflower Mash

This is *serious* comfort food!

SERVES 1

1 cauliflower head
   (typically 200g)
1 small chicken breast
   (typically 125g)
1 small handful grated
   Cheddar (approx. 30g)
1 level tsp butter (approx. 10g)

1 Preheat the oven to 200°C/fan 180°C.

2 Bring a pan of salted water to the boil and add the cauliflower. Reduce the heat and simmer for 20–30 minutes.

3 Season the chicken breast with salt and pepper, and roast uncovered in the oven for 20–30 minutes, or until the juices run clear.

4 Remove the chicken from the oven and sprinkle with the cheese, then return it to the oven for a final 5–10 minutes, until the cheese is melted.

5 Meanwhile, drain the cauliflower and return it to the pan. Season with salt and pepper, add the butter and mash well.

6 Spoon the cauliflower on to a plate and place the chicken on top. Season again and serve.

Chicken Sausages and Cheesy Broccoli Mash

The star of the show! A new take on the original Body Blitz classic!

SERVES 1

2 chicken sausages
   (typically 34g each)
   (Heck Chicken Chipolatas
   are my favourite)
1 small broccoli head
   (typically 200g), broken
   into florets
1 level tsp butter (approx. 10g)
1 small handful grated
   Cheddar (approx. 30g)
1 tsp Heinz Reduced Salt and
   Sugar Ketchup (optional)

1 Preheat the grill to medium-high.

2 Bring a large pan of salted water to the boil and add the broccoli florets. Reduce the heat and simmer for 20–30 minutes, until tender.

3 Pierce the sausages with a fork and grill for 15 minutes, turning occasionally, until cooked through.

4 Drain the broccoli and return it to the pan. Season with salt and pepper, add the butter and mash.

5 Spoon the broccoli mash into the centre of a plate, place the sausages on top and sprinkle with the Cheddar. Drizzle with ketchup, if using, to serve.

Chicken and Prawn Hot and Sour Soup

This is nice and warming on a cold day!

SERVES 1

1 tsp sesame oil

1 tsp finely chopped garlic

½ red chilli, finely chopped

1 small chicken breast (typically 125g), chopped into small pieces

1 large handful button mushrooms (approx. 100g), halved

1 small packet raw prawns (typically 150g)

1 large handful spinach

½ chicken stock cube

400ml boiling water

1 tbsp soy sauce

juice of ½ lime

1 Place the oil, garlic and chilli in a large, deep frying pan or wok and place over a medium–high heat. When the oil starts spitting, add the chicken and cook for 2–3 minutes.

2 Add the mushrooms and continue to fry until the chicken is cooked and the mushrooms have softened.

3 Stir in the prawns and toss all ingredients together, until the prawns are cooked through.

4 Dissolve the chicken stock cube in the water then add this to the pan with the spinach, followed by the soy sauce and lime juice. Season with salt and pepper to taste and serve.

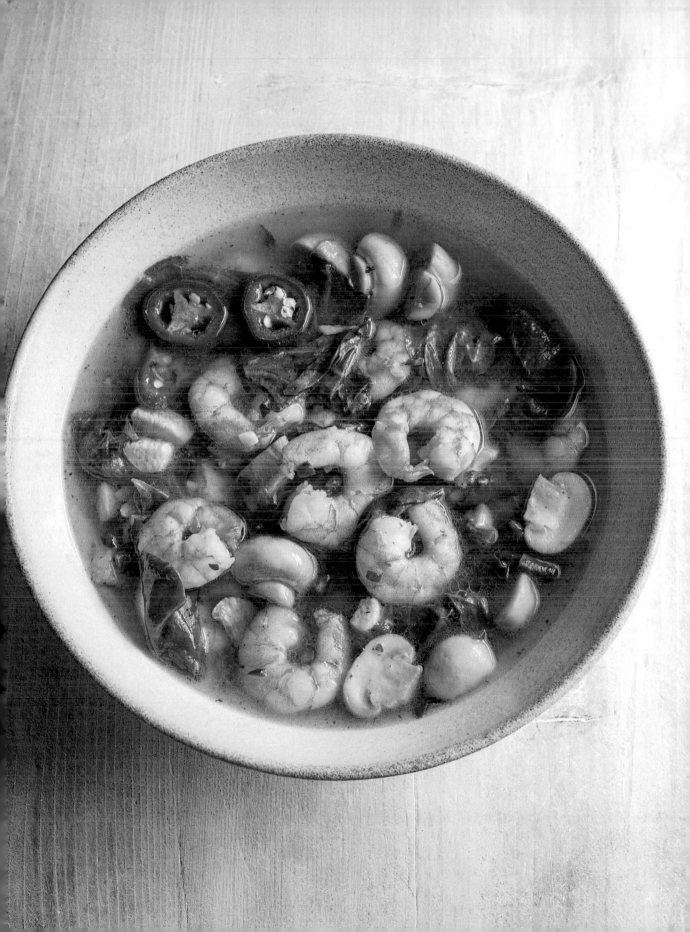

Prawn and Feta Tapas Bowl

I had this at a hotel in Florida when I was
a teenager and I've been making it ever since!

SERVES 1

1 tsp olive oil
½ small white onion, diced
1 small packet raw prawns
(typically 150g)
½ × 400g tin chopped
tomatoes
1 small handful cubed feta
(approx. 30g)
1 large handful spinach and/
or rocket and/or lettuce,
to serve

1 Place the oil in a frying pan over a medium–
high heat.

2 Add the onion to the pan, stir and cook for
4–5 minutes, or until soft.

3 Add the prawns and toss in the pan for
2–3 minutes, until pink and cooked through.

4 Lower the heat, stir in the chopped tomatoes
and simmer for 5 minutes.

5 Finally, crumble in the feta and leave to melt.

6 Season with salt and pepper to taste and
serve alongside the salad leaves.

Fats Stacked Turkey Burger

The carb free *and* lean burger option! Try seasoning the burger with a pinch of dried oregano, some chopped fresh parsley or even a dash of Worcestershire sauce.

SERVES 1

100g turkey breast mince
1 whole egg
1 small red onion, peeled and
    ½ diced and ½ finely sliced
your choice of herbs/spices/
    seasoning
1 spray Fry Light cooking
    spray (optional)
1 slice halloumi
    (typically 30g)
1 large handful spinach and/
    or rocket
1 lettuce leaf
½ small tomato, finely sliced
1 pickle, finely sliced
1 tsp Heinz Reduced Salt and
    Sugar Ketchup (optional)

1 Combine the mince, egg, diced onion and chosen seasoning together in a bowl. Mould and flatten the mixture into a burger.

2 Place a small frying pan over a medium heat and spray with Fry Light, if using. Add the turkey burger to the pan, sear on each side, then fry for about 5 minutes on each side, or until cooked through.

3 Place the halloumi in the pan next to the burger and allow to melt slightly.

4 Arrange the handful of spinach or rocket leaves on a plate and top with the turkey burger and halloumi. Place the lettuce leaf, tomato, sliced onion and pickle on top of the burger and drizzle with ketchup, if using, to serve

Chicken Pesto Courgetti

This is how I make a low-carb version of my favourite pasta dish.

SERVES 1

1 small chicken breast
(typically 125g)
1 large courgette
(typically 250–300g)
1 level tbsp any pesto
(approx. 15g)
1 level tbsp pine nuts
(approx. 15g)
1 large handful rocket
2 level tbsp finely grated
Parmesan (approx. 20g)

1 Preheat the oven to 200°C/fan 180°C.

2 Season the chicken breast and bake uncovered for 20–30 minutes, or until the juices run clear.

3 Meanwhile, grate the courgetti into long strands (vertically down the largest slicing option on a cheese grater will do the trick – or you could use a spiraliser).

4 Place the courgetti in a saucepan over a medium heat, season with salt and pepper, and cook for 3–4 minutes.

5 Remove the chicken from oven and, using 2 forks, shred the meat before adding it to the courgetti.

6 Stir in the pesto and pine nuts and check the seasoning.

7 Serve on a bed of rocket with Parmesan scattered over the top.

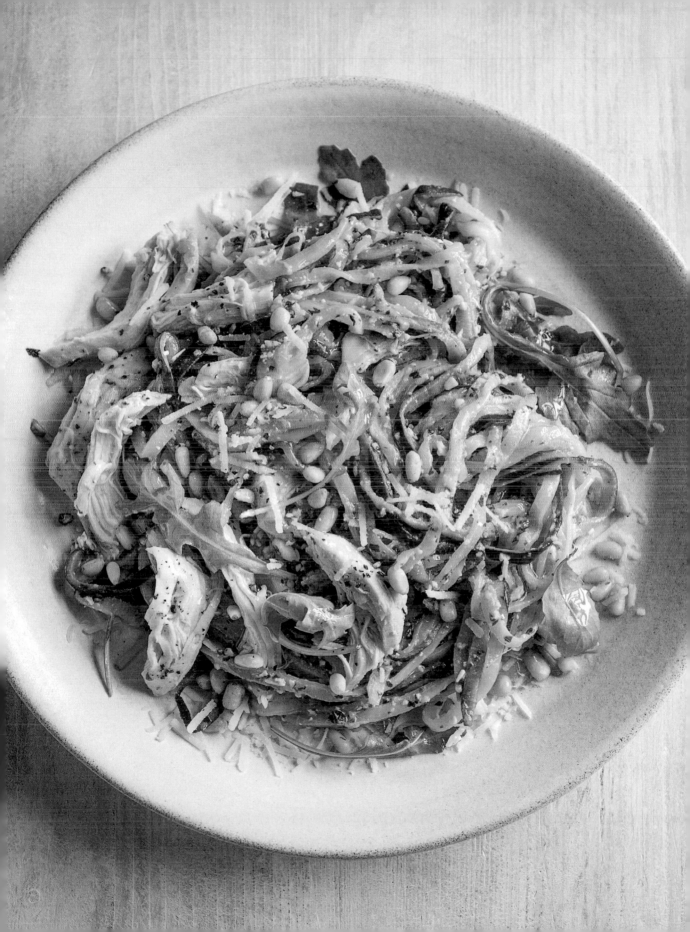

Spicy Beef Lettuce Wraps

Learn to replace carbs with veg in every which way and life gets *a lot* easier! You could try adding a little ground cumin and coriander to the mince.

SERVES 1

1 spray Fry Light cooking spray (optional)
125g 5% beef mince
your choice of herbs/spices/hot sauce
½ tomato, diced
½ white onion, peeled and diced
½ jalapeño pepper, diced
juice of ½ lime
2–4 large lettuce leaves
1 large handful grated Cheddar (approx. 30g)

1 Place a small frying pan over a medium–high heat and spray with Fry Light, if using. Add the mince and your choice of seasoning and brown for 5–10 minutes, until cooked through.

2 Meanwhile, combine the tomato, onion, jalapeño and lime juice in a bowl to make a salsa.

3 Place the lettuce leaves on a serving plate and divide the cooked mince between them. Sprinkle them with cheese, top with the salsa and serve.

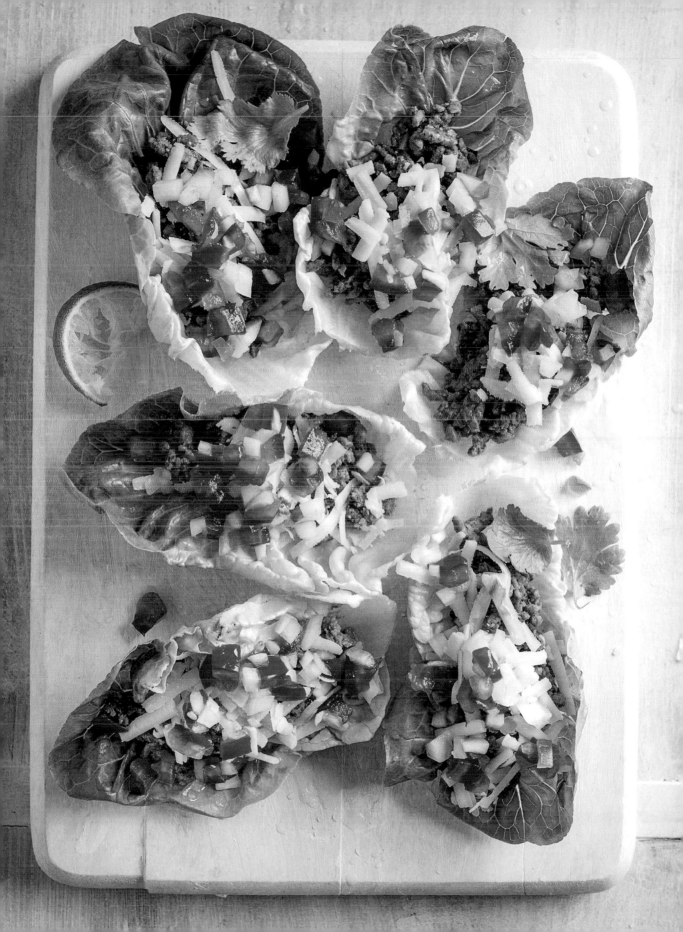

TRACKING YOUR PROGRESS

Let me state right now that you absolutely *do not* have to track your progress.

However, for some people, tracking can be a *great* way of holding oneself accountable and congratulating oneself when all is said and done.

I say *when all is said and done* because even though you *might* see progress weekly, you *might not*.

Weight loss, fat loss, body transformation – this is *not* a linear process.

It is a bumpy ride full of results and plateaus, energy and lethargy, hunger and satiety.

Trust me when I say that no single day or week will feel or look the same.

Some people lose weight and/or inches week on week for a substantial amount of time (usually complete beginners to diet and exercise) but most of us do not. For most of us (myself included), results can happen substantially one week and halt completely the next. They can be gradual and seem insignificant (until the end), or they can come in huge peaks and frustrating troughs.

Everybody is Different

It goes without saying that if you are a size 10, your weight loss is not going to be nearly as substantial as somebody who is coming in as a size 18.

However, this success can be flipped in a different context.

A size 10's before and after photos could look, on the surface of things and to the untrained eye, much more impressive than a size 18's. This is simply because the size 10 is starting at a substantially lower overall body fat percentage, so where they end up could be the ultimate end goal for many of us.

This may all sound very callous but, having done this for six years, I speak from experience when I say – progress will look and feel different for *everybody*.

Having said all that, if you do want to track your progress, here's how to do it...

Those of you who have the original book will know this well, but have a read anyway to refresh your Blitzer brain!

Weighing In

>> Make a note of your weight on morning one of your fat-loss plan with no food or water in your system.

Then weigh in this way again:

>> As many mornings a week as you wish (but be prepared to see the scale jump around if you weigh yourself very regularly) OR
>> Once a week until the last day of your fat-loss plan

If your plan involves a carb cycle:

>> Weigh in *before* your re-feed days as well as *after* your re-feed days

Re-feeds *affect* everybody differently – some will lose after and some will gain after. This is all to do with water and carbohydrate storage in the body, it is *not* to do with body fat gain and loss (hence the Saturday *and* Monday weigh-ins to get a more accurate idea of where you stand).

Please remember that:

>> Fibre (veg and most 'diet foods')
>> Menstrual cycle (hormones and water retention)
>> Water intake (more or less than usual)
>> Carb cycling (overall food intake and glycogen storage)
>> Stress (both physical and mental)
>> Lack of sleep (cortisol levels)
>> Sodium (salt intake)

will *all* affect your weigh-ins.

This is why *some* people feel that more frequent weigh-ins allow for more accurate tracking, while others feel that they create only more confusion. Honestly, it all depends on the type of person you are.

I weigh-in most days when in a fat-loss phase, as it gives me a more accurate assessment of my progress and my body's response to food, water and hormonal changes.

However frequently you decide to weigh in, if you *do* see the scales acting erratically, remember the list of factors that affect your weigh-ins, take a deep breath and stay calm.

Body Fat %

I do not advocate body-fat measurements by machine, as I have yet to see an accurate reading from anything other than an ultrasound.

If you are interested in tracking your own Body Fat %, though, I suggest you take measurements using callipers. You can buy BF callipers online – simply follow the instructions that come with them. Alternatively, ask a PT or GP to do this for you.

Measurements

Like weighing in, measurements can sometimes be misleading. I say this because newbies *at the very beginning* of their fitness journey can find that while they can lose 1cm of fat rapidly, they can also gain 1cm of muscle rapidly. However, *for most people*, measurements are still a great way to track progress.

The most important measurement to track is your waist, as that is the least likely place to gain muscle. You should measure the rest of the body but, if the results are erratic, remember that your waist is the best area to judge fat-loss progress.

>> Using a material measuring tape, make a note of the following measurements on day 1 of your fat-loss plan with no food or water in your system:

1. **Chest:** Measure all the way around your chest at its broadest
2. **Waist:** Measure all the way around your waist at its narrowest
3. **Hips:** Measure all the way around your hips at their widest
4. **Thighs:** Measure all the way around one upper leg at its widest
5. **Arms:** Measure all the way around one upper arm at its widest

>> Take these measurements once a fortnight, first thing in the morning with no food or water in your system

Progress Pics

My personal favourite...

I recommend taking progress pics no more than once a fortnight. I say this because aesthetic results take time to appear, and you will probably feel disheartened with a week 1/week 2 comparison.

>> Take the following pictures (ideally in daylight) on day 1 of your fat-loss plan with no food or water in your system:

1. **Front on**
2. **Side on**
3. **From behind (if possible)**

Take the pictures again on day 15 of your fat-loss plan with no food or water in your system. Finally, take them on day 29 of your fat-loss plan with no food or water in your system.

If you have followed the plan 100% and you compare your day 1 and day 29 images side by side, I have every confidence that you will be amazed.

A FINAL WORD...

I hope that this book has helped you find a way to incorporate exercise and nutrition into your life.

If you've finished one of the 4-week plans and you'd like to continue, then please do so. You can do any of the plans in this book for up to 24 weeks (6 months). Feel free to move on to the next plan, or stick to the same one, whatever suits you best.

At the 24-week point, though, I suggest you *slowly and gradually* come out of the calorie deficit instructed in the plan

I'd like you to do this via *both* your food intake (ideally with a gradual, weekly carb increase) *and* your training output.

When coming out of a deficit, I typically:

>> Add 1 high-carb snack or meal to my daily intake each week, until I have full days of higher calories and balanced meals of protein, carbs and fats.

>> Reduce my training by 1–2 days weekly and/or slowly and gradually reduce my cardio time (by, say, 10 minutes weekly), until I feel I have reached a happy balance of fun training days and total rest days.

I would never encourage somebody to push their body for longer than a few months at a time but, equally, I wouldn't encourage somebody to under-exercise and/or overeat.

I find that 3 full rest days and 1 full day of dietary freedom a week is as comfortable as it gets.

That's not to say I restrict my food every day – I certainly do *not* diet all year round! But I don't throw myself into takeaway Mecca either. And neither should you, because that leads to a never-ending cycle of playing cat and mouse with your body *and* your brain.

Please feel free to follow me on social media (@madeleychloe), visit my blog where I talk about all of this in detail (fitnessfondue.com) and keep me updated with your thoughts, questions and progress.

Until next time, Blitzers!

INDEX

ACKNOWLEDGEMENTS

First and foremost, I want to thank every single Body Blitzer who
bought the first book and made it possible for me to write a second...
THANK YOU!
Six years ago, I had a few hundred followers and a handful of clients, and
my dream was one day to help thousands of women around the world
change their lives. Thanks to you guys, I watch this dream take more vivid
shape every year. I am so grateful for your continued trust and support.

I also want to thank my amazing agent, Clare Hulton, who bought
into my dream from day one and never once made me compromise it.
Thank you for working your little socks off for me, Clare!

Next to my INCREDIBLY TALENTED team at Transworld!
Michelle, Becky, Emma – you are the absolute dream team and
I am SO LUCKY that I get to work with you for another year!

To Jo Roberts-Miller and Emma and Alex Smith, thank you for making
this book look so beautiful and for staying up until sunrise to make sure that
the crazy control freak inside my head was happy. You are so amazingly
talented and I am so very grateful for your daily grind on this book!

Sam Riley and Meerah Shah, I am SO happy I found you both!
These long, gruelling shoot days would be a total schlep without you
two there to play with, and lord knows I would not look as fresh!
May we be doing this together forever more!

All the equipment I used in the photos is by PULSE FITNESS. If you are
interested in purchasing any fitness equipment whatsoever (from a mat,
to a dumbbell, or even a Smith machine) for your home or gym, Pulse
can provide, deliver and set up your desired space. You can find them at:
http://thepulsegroup.co.uk/pulse-fitness

Lastly, to my fiancé James...
I think you have seen me have more meltdowns this year than ever before!
Redecorating, wedding planning, editing one book and writing another
all in the space of a few short months was... interesting... but every time
you held my little melted head you made me love you even more.
Thank you.
I am so excited to marry you.